Advanced Clinical Practice in Healthcare

This book outlines the key components of advanced clinical practice, with new and expanded practice elements added to this fully updated second edition. It discusses vital issues for providing effective evidence-based healthcare, emphasising the role that advanced practice has to play in contemporary healthcare provision.

Throughout the book, new ways of thinking and implementing changes in relation to practice, education and research are described. Divided into three sections with the addition of a newly revised introduction and a review of the evolution of advanced practice, this book covers:

- The provision of guidance on the development and implementation of clinical skills, including consultation, clinical decision making, holistic care and the role of care planning in advanced practice.
- The explanation of management skills and how to manage in this changing healthcare environment. It also explains how to negotiate and monitor the complexities of the present and changing healthcare system to ensure delivery of quality patient care.
- The clarification of the professional role of the advanced practice clinician and how implementation of the role can influence and improve the delivery of patient care.

Case studies and activities that assist in the development, implementation and extension of advanced practice are included in each chapter.

This book is particularly relevant to advanced practice clinicians including nurses, midwives and allied health professionals practising within primary and secondary care. It is designed for those who wish to further advance their practice, to clarify their roles within the context of advanced practice and to prepare for future roles that will have significant implications for patient care delivery, improved patient outcomes and patient satisfaction.

Carol L. Cox is Professor Emeritus, City St. George's University of London, London, England; Philosophy, Sociology and Theology/Religion Teacher at Pensacola Catholic High School, Pensacola, Florida, USA and Volunteer Registered Nurse at the Health and Hope Clinic, Pensacola, Florida, USA.

Marie C. Hill is Associate Professor (Practice Nursing) City St. George's, University of London, England and Programme Director MSc/PgDip (Primary Care Practice Nursing).

Victoria M. Lack is an Advanced Nurse Practitioner (Urgent Care) at Mid Yorkshire NHS Teaching Trust, UK and a Teacher in Advanced Clinical Practice.

"It is a pleasure to endorse this book on Advanced Practice. Clearly, the world of advanced practice is changing which articulates the need for new perspectives on advanced practice and its implementation in the clinical environment. We now see new arenas of practice for the advanced practice nurse, midwife and allied health professional. No longer can we rely on old narratives and old practices. Excitingly, this second edition addresses new perspectives and recommendations for practice. It is evident that healthcare is evolving rapidly. This book will assist you in keeping abreast of changes occurring today and tomorrow. Read this book. It will make a difference in your thinking and your practice."

B. Rieland, MSc, APRN, *Chief Clinical Officer, Health and Hope Clinic, Pensacola, Florida*

Advanced Clinical Practice in Healthcare

Changing and Evolving Clinical Roles for Nurses and Allied Health Professionals

Second edition

Edited by Carol L. Cox, Marie C. Hill and Victoria M. Lack

Routledge
Taylor & Francis Group
LONDON AND NEW YORK

Designed cover image: Getty Images

Second edition published 2027
by Routledge
4 Park Square, Milton Park, Abingdon, Oxon, OX14 4RN

and by Routledge
605 Third Avenue, New York, NY 10158

Routledge is an imprint of the Taylor & Francis Group, an informa business

First edition published by Routledge 2011

British Library Cataloguing-in-Publication Data
A catalogue record for this book is available from the British Library

Library of Congress Cataloging-in-Publication Data
Names: Cox, Carol Lynn editor | Hill, Marie C. (Marie Catherine),
1959– editor | Lack, Victoria M. editor
Title: Advanced clinical practice in healthcare : changing and evolving
clinical roles for nurses and allied health professionals /
[edited by Carol Cox, Marie Hill, Victoria Lack].
Other titles: Advanced practice in healthcare
Description: Second edition. | Abingdon, Oxon ; New York, NY :
Routledge, 2026. | Includes bibliographical references and index.
Identifiers: LCCN 2026023552 (print) | LCCN 2026023553 (ebook) |
ISBN 9781041002901 hbk | ISBN 9781041002758 pbk | ISBN 9781003609049 ebk
Subjects: LCSH: Nursing | Allied health personnel
Classification: LCC RT82 .A37 2026 (print) | LCC RT82 (ebook)
LC record available at https://lccn.loc.gov/2026023552
LC ebook record available at https://lccn.loc.gov/2026023553

ISBN: 9781041002901 (hbk)
ISBN: 9781041002758 (pbk)
ISBN: 9781003609049 (ebk)

DOI: 10.4324/9781003609049

Typeset in Sabon
by Newgen Publishing UK

To Jim, Colin and Pete.
Thank you for all of your support.

Contents

About the Editors

Carol L. Cox, PhD, MA, MSc, MA, PG Dip, BA (Hons), BSc (Hons), RN, FHEA, OP Professor Emeritus, City St George's, University of London, London, England, UK. Volunteer Registered Nurse, Health and Hope Clinic, Pensacola, Florida, USA.

Marie C. Hill, PhD, MHM, PG Dip, BSc (Hons), SFHEA, RN, Associate Professor (Practice Nursing), Department of Nursing and Midwifery, School of Health & Medical Sciences (Clerkenwell Campus) City St. George's, University of London, London, England, UK.

Victoria M. Lack, MSc (Family Nurse Practitioner), MSc (Tropical and Infectious Disease), PG Dip, BNurs (Hons), RGN ANP (Urgent Care) Mid Yorkshire Teaching NHS Trust, UK. Teacher (Advanced Clinical Practice).

Contributors

Foreword: **Helen Gibbons**, MSc, NMC Teacher, BA (Hons), RN, FHEA, Lead Nurse (England and Northern Ireland), RCN King's Nursing Cadets, Institute of Nursing Excellence, Royal College of Nursing, London, England, UK, www.rcn.org.uk
Endorsement: Bonnie Rieland, MSc, APRN, Chief Clinical Officer, Health and Hope Clinic, Pensacola, Florida.

Siobhan Hicks, MSc, PG Cert (Leadership), PG Cert (Academic Practice), BSc (Hons), NP Diploma Practice Nursing, RGN
Interim Co Director of Nursing, Bromley By Bow Health Partnership (bbbc.org.uk)
Clinical Lead (Primary Care, Network 6) Bromley by Bow and Stepney Health CIC
Advanced Nurse Practitioner General Practice.

Jane Sumner, PhD, MSc, BSN, Dip N, RN, APRN, BC
Professor Emeritus, Louisiana State University Health Sciences Center School of Nursing
New Orleans, Louisiana, USA.

Kathryn Waddington, PhD, MSc, BSc
Emerita Fellow in Psychology and Chartered Coaching Psychologist
School of Social Sciences
University of Westminster, London.

Ruth Walters, MSc, BA (Hons), RGN (Inactive)
Advanced Nurse Practitioner and Diabetes Nurse Specialist,
Primary Care (Retired).

Nicola Whiteing, PhD, RN
Associate Professor, Chair of Discipline Allied Health, Midwifery & Community
Southern Cross University, New South Wales, Australia.

Foreword

Sir Jonathan Asbridge, when he was President of the Nursing and Midwifery Council, wrote the Foreword for the first edition of *Advanced Practice in Healthcare*, skills for nurses and allied health professionals. A decade later, much of what he predicted has occurred. With the advent of new roles for advanced practice practitioners, for example, Pharmacists assessing, diagnosing and prescribing, it is clear there is pressure to keep up with the pace of change. Furthermore, Artificial Intelligence (AI) can aid in your assessment, diagnosis and decision making when making use of new technologies. Based on the knowledge this book provides you can discern when to use AI and when not. By gaining the knowledge articulated in the second edition of *Advanced Practice in Healthcare* you can acquire new ways to think about patient care issues and how to manage patient expectations associated with their problems. Keep in mind that this book will also provide guidance on how to hone your skills to ensure you are an expert who influences the delivery of clinically effective care.

Being and remaining at the forefront of healthcare delivery requires knowledge in clinical decision making, consultation techniques and sound care planning. It also requires knowing how to be an effective manager. One who is able to manage situations and others as an advanced practitioner as well as lead and influence others. Your challenge is and will continue to be remaining insightful so that you can keep abreast of the rapidly changing landscape. Never before have such significant changes occurred within the healthcare system. As Sir Asbridge wrote, "Advanced Practice in Healthcare is an insightful book that addresses the knowledge and skills advanced practitioners must master in order to lead these changes." This second edition contains new and expansive knowledge that will guide you towards the goals you want to achieve.

Helen Gibbons, MSc, NMC Teacher, BA (Hons), RN, FHEA
Lead Nurse (England and Northern Ireland)
RCN King's Nursing Cadets
Institute of Nursing Excellence
Royal College of Nursing
London, England, UK
www.rcn.org.uk

Preface

The first edition of *Advanced Practice in Healthcare,* skills for nurses and allied health professionals was written for aspiring advanced-level practitioners. In this second edition, information has been updated and extended not only for the aspiring advanced-level practitioner, but also for seasoned advanced-level practitioners who wish to obtain updated information about what advanced-level practice is now, and how their professions are evolving. Without question, the advanced level of care provided by these practitioners is emerging in new arenas. The landscape in healthcare has changed and is continuing to change and evolve. Therefore, the skills and knowledge for advanced practice are broadening rapidly. This is seen in healthcare delivery by filling critical gaps in physician shortages, such as critical care practitioners in intensive care and primary providers in urgent care, accident and emergency rooms and primary care. These practitioners are, by their very nature, increasing patient access, especially in rural/underserved areas, improving continuity of care through team-based models and taking on broader responsibilities in primary, specialty and hospital settings. There is projected growth within the advanced-level disciplines far exceeding the average for other occupations. This expansion involves greater autonomy (Full Practice Authority in many states in the United States of America and delegated 'Full' Practice Authority in General Practice and some Firms in the United Kingdom). Integration into all levels of healthcare, and formalised structures for professional growth, driven by demand for cost-effective, comprehensive care, is seen as never before. Expansion drivers are subsequent to physician shortages and generalist expertise needed in primary care and acute care (e.g. in acute medicine; surgical services; anaesthesia; women's and men's health and midwifery) and where there is an increased demand for services relating to the increasing ageing population and chronic disease management, for example, in rural areas, home health care and geriatric services. Practice in these areas is increasingly becoming without physician oversight. Reliance on advanced-level practitioners has become essential in the provision of accessible high-quality care. In addition, these practitioners are employed to manage patient loads, reduce waiting times and offer personalised care (e.g., counselling and mental health services). Their service is cost-effective as they improve efficiency and reduce costs by lowering unnecessary accident and emergency room visits and hospitalisations.

In this second edition you will learn about this and much more. For example, you will learn about the broader scope of advanced practice, how advanced-level practitioners diagnose, treat, prescribe, manage more complex heath conditions and work collaboratively and independently. Growth has never been stronger in areas like improving access to care and promotion of better health through patient-centred care with an emphasis on patient education. You will also learn how advanced-level practitioners are taking on positions in leadership, education and management. Excitingly, you will see in this second edition that advanced-level practitioners are shaping healthcare delivery and the future of nursing and allied health professionals.

In this book there are illuminating perspectives on where advanced-level practice emerged as a discipline and the formation of new thinking and world views. For example, this book begins by articulating the history of nursing with its changes in context and evolution to today's advanced-level practice. It also presents projections for the future.

The introduction to our Chapter 1, From the beginning to advanced practice: An *expanded historical narrative* provides the context for the development of advanced practice both in the United States of America and in the United Kingdom. The second edition is then divided into three discrete sections.

In Part 1, Chapter 2 addresses consultation skills by examining several models of consultation, as well as practical ways to enable a successful consultation, to ensure the best possible outcomes for the patient and clinician. There is an opportunity to reflect on changes in methods of consultation and how this can affect practice both now and in the future. Chapter 3 considers the key steps involved in clinical decision making, and how knowledge and skills can be applied to facilitate this process. Clinical governance and supervision are also discussed, as decision making is not only the responsibility of the individual practitioner. Chapter 4 discusses the care planning process and its direction and delivery by advanced-level practitioners. Specific skills are identified as required for successful care planning which are crucial to enable holistic and realistic care in practice.

In Part 2, Chapter 5 articulates management in terms of its definition and how management theories have developed and evolved. This chapter explores how management theories have influenced and are influencing today's healthcare delivery systems. The diverse role of the manager is explored as well as strategies that managers use to enhance their role. Chapter 6 explores the concept of emotional intelligence (EI) and emotional quotient (EQ). It identifies ways in which emotional intelligence principles can be applied to management practice. This chapter explores communication and management skills, facilitated by reflective practice. Thus, enabling an opportunity to identify management skills and areas for development. Chapter 7 examines the role of the advanced-level practitioner in the United States of America. It explicates the levels of education required and how the education landscape has changed from master's-level to doctoral-level education. It illuminates different specialties of advanced practice in nursing and the organisations that influence advanced-level education, accreditation, certification and practice. It also delineates lessons learned during the Covid-19 pandemic and how these are influencing nursing education.

In Part 3, various aspects of leadership and the professional role are examined. Chapter 8 describes the elements of professionalism in advanced-level practice. It considers and explores professionalism from its broadest perspective in clinical and direct care. The changing arena of practice is addressed as well as how the constructs of professionalism influence all aspects of advanced-level practice. Chapter 9 provides background information relating to clinical effectiveness and its importance in shaping patient outcomes. It presents ways to become involved as a case manager in influencing the implementation of evidence-based practice and provides guidance on instruments/tools that can be utilised to review practice. Finally, there is consideration for ways in which the advanced practitioner can address continuing professional development activities for the benefit of the organisation and their own self-development. Part 3 concludes with Chapter 10 which explores the value and benefits of coaching to promote advanced practice, leadership development and interprofessional collaborative practice in healthcare teams. As well as understanding the psychology of leadership, this chapter considers the relevance of systems-psychodynamic thinking and coaching to help recognise and address unconscious dynamics, processes and defences in individuals, teams and organisations. There are opportunities to critically reflect upon influencing skills, assumptions and ability to lead and manage with political awareness.

The authors that have contributed to this book are experts in the field of advanced-level practice. Each chapter has been written with the intention of advancing and extending your practice as well as preparing you for what is to come in advanced-level practice. Beyond the enjoyment of reading this book, it is postulated your eyes will become open to new and innovative ways to develop yourself and develop your career in advanced-level practice.

Carol L. Cox, Marie C. Hill and Victoria M. Lack

Introduction

Carol L. Cox, Marie C. Hill and Victoria M. Lack

When we undertook the endeavor to write with colleagues the first edition of *Advanced Practice in Healthcare*, Skills for nurses and allied health professionals, we envisioned it would influence practice. However, we did not see the significant impact it would have on advanced practice clinicians/practitioners' ways of thinking and influencing patient care. A decade on, what was predicted in the first edition has come to fruition. Now we stand on the precipice of a new era of advanced practice. One that has immense significance for how patient care is managed and delivered. In this second edition we have constructed an extension to the first edition. It takes the practitioner beyond the boundaries of practice, viewed by many as constrained by traditional boundaries, to what is happening in practice now and forward into the future of practice.

Advanced practice entails a transformative evolution in healthcare delivery. It extends beyond traditional nursing boundaries to encompass independent clinical decision-making, diagnostic capabilities, and comprehensive patient management (Bales et al, 2025). The role of Advanced Practice Clinicians/Practitioners has fundamentally reshaped how patient care is conceptualized and delivered across diverse healthcare arenas. This book explores the essential dimensions of advanced clinical practice, including core competencies, scope of practice, and the evolving landscape of these critical roles in modern healthcare systems.

Core competencies of advanced practice clinicians

Advanced practice clinicians operate within a well-defined framework of competencies that have distinguished their practice as different than traditional nursing/practitioner roles. The Hamric & Hanson model establishes six foundational competencies that guide advanced practice (Bales et al, 2025; Schlunegger et al, 2021). These are:

- Direct Clinical Practice: forms the cornerstone of advanced practice, encompassing comprehensive assessment, diagnosis, and management of acute and chronic

DOI: 10.4324/9781003609049-1

conditions. This competency requires advanced knowledge and clinical judgment to evaluate complex patient presentations and determine appropriate interventions.
- Guidance and Coaching: involves educating patients and families about health conditions, treatment options, and self-management strategies. Advanced practice clinicians facilitate informed decision-making and empower patients to actively participate in their care plans (Bales et al, 2025)
- Evidence-Based Practice: mandates that clinical decisions be grounded in current research, clinical expertise, and patient preferences. Advanced practice clinicians synthesize evidence to improve outcomes and contribute to the advancement of clinical knowledge (Bales et al, 2025)
- Leadership: extends beyond individual patient care to influence organizational policies, quality improvement initiatives, and healthcare system development. Advanced practice clinicians advocate for patients and drive systemic changes that enhance care delivery (Bales et al, 2025 Schlunegger et al, 2021).
- Collaboration: requires effective communication and partnership with interdisciplinary healthcare teams, including physicians, social workers, pharmacists, and other specialists. This competency ensures coordinated, comprehensive care across multiple providers (Bales et al, 2025 Schlunegger et al, 2021).
- Ethical Decision-Making: demands that advanced practice clinicians navigate complex moral dilemmas with integrity, applying ethical frameworks to resolve conflicts between patient autonomy, beneficence, and organizational constraints (Schlunegger et al, 2021).

These competencies are addressed in this book with an emphasis on scope of practice now and as predicted in the future.

Scope of practice

The scope of practice for advanced practice clinicians encompasses a comprehensive range of clinical activities that vary by setting, specialization, and regulatory jurisdiction (Bales et al, 2025, Sondergaard et al, 2024, Schlunegger et al, 2021). The Scope of Practice involves:

- Assessment and Diagnosis: includes conducting detailed health histories, performing physical examinations, ordering and interpreting diagnostic tests, and formulating differential diagnoses. Advanced practice clinicians synthesize clinical data to identify underlying health problems and determine appropriate diagnostic pathways (Sondergaard et al, 2024).
- Pharmacological Management: permits advanced practice clinicians to prescribe medications, adjust dosages, and monitor therapeutic responses. This authority varies by state and country but generally includes both controlled and non-controlled substances within their specialty area (Bales et al, 2025, Schlunegger et al, 2021).
- Care Coordination: involves organizing and managing patient care across multiple providers and settings. Advanced practice clinicians serve as care coordinators in integrated care models, particularly for patients with multimorbid conditions requiring complex management (Bales et al, 2025).

- Counseling and Patient Education: extends beyond basic health teaching to include motivational interviewing, behavioral modification strategies, and psychosocial support. These interventions promote health literacy and facilitate patient engagement in self-management (Bales et al, 2025, Sondergaard et al, 2024, Schlunegger et al, 2021).
- Management of Acute and Chronic Conditions: encompasses the full spectrum of clinical care, from acute illness management in hospital settings to chronic disease management in primary care and specialty clinics. Advanced practice clinicians provide continuity of care and long-term disease management (Bales et al, 2025, Sondergaard, et al 2024).

Evolution over the past decade

The past decade has witnessed significant expansion and refinement of advanced practice roles. These have been driven by healthcare system demands and considerable research evidence that demonstrates improved patient outcomes (Bales et al, 2025, Sondergaard, et al 2024). The evolution is seen in:

- Integration into Multimorbidity Care Models represents a major evolution, with advanced practice clinicians increasingly leading care for patients with multiple concurrent chronic conditions. This shift reflects recognition that complex patients benefit from the holistic, systems-level approach characteristic of advanced practice (Bales et al, 2025).
- Emphasis on Leadership and Systems-Level Impact has grown exponentially, with advanced practice clinicians moving beyond bedside care to influence organizational strategy, quality metrics, and healthcare policy. This evolution acknowledges that advanced practice clinicians are positioned to bridge clinical and administrative perspectives (Bales et al, 2025, Sondergaard et al, 2024).
- Regulatory and Scope Expansion has occurred in many jurisdictions, though barriers remain in regions with restrictive regulations (particularly in the United Kingdom). In the main, progressive healthcare systems have expanded independent practice authority for advanced practice clinicians, recognizing their capacity for autonomous clinical decision-making (Bales et al, 2025)
- Evidence-Based Model Development has accelerated, with research increasingly documenting the effectiveness of Advanced Practice Nursing (APN)-led interventions, care models, and outcomes. This evidence base supports continued expansion of advanced practice roles and informs best practice standards (Bales et al, 2025, Sondergaard et al, 2024).

Current trends in advanced practice

Contemporary advanced practice is characterized by several significant trends that shape current practice and forecast future directions (Bales et al, 2025, Sondergaard et al, 2024). These are seen as:

- APN-Led Care Models are demonstrating improved patient outcomes, enhanced self-management, and increased health literacy. These models position advanced practice clinicians as primary providers, particularly in primary care, chronic disease management, and specialty clinics (Bales et al, 2025, Sondergaard et al, 2024).

- Person-Centered Care Integration emphasizes individualized treatment plans that respect patient values, preferences, and cultural contexts. Advanced practice clinicians increasingly employ shared decision-making frameworks and incorporate patient-reported outcomes into clinical practice (Sondergaard et al, 2024).
- Collaborative Practice Structures reflect recognition that optimal patient outcomes demand interdisciplinary teamwork. Advanced practice clinicians function as full team members, contributing specialized expertise while respecting the contributions of other healthcare professionals (Bales et al, 2025, Sondergaard et al, 2024).
- Academic and Research Engagement has expanded, with advanced practice clinicians increasingly involved in clinical research, quality improvement projects, and scholarly activities. This engagement strengthens the evidence base for advanced practice and contributes to professional development (Sondergaard et al, 2024).
- Technology Integration facilitates remote monitoring, telehealth delivery, and data-driven decision-making. Advanced practice clinicians leverage technology to extend access to care and enhance clinical efficiency (Bales et al, 2025).

Advanced practice versus traditional nursing

While advanced practice clinicians have emerged from nursing backgrounds, their practice differs fundamentally from traditional nursing roles in scope, authority, and impact (Bales et al, 2025, Sondergaard et al, 2024, Thomas et al, 2012). This is seen primarily in areas such as:

- Independent Diagnosis and Decision-Making represent the most significant distinction. Advanced practice clinicians formulate independent diagnoses and make autonomous clinical decisions, whereas traditional nurses implement care plans designed by physicians or other providers (Schulunegger et al, 2024, Thomas et al, 2012).
- Holistic Patient Management extends beyond symptom management to encompass comprehensive disease management, preventive care, and health promotion. Advanced practice clinicians address the full spectrum of patient health needs rather than specific nursing interventions (Sondergaard et al, 2024, Schulunegger et al, 2024, Thomas et al, 2012).
- Systems-Level Impact distinguishes advanced practice from traditional nursing. Advanced practice clinicians influence organizational policies, care models, and healthcare systems, whereas traditional nursing focuses primarily on individual patient care and unit-level operations (Schulunegger et al, 2024, Thomas et al, 2012).
- Prescriptive Authority permits advanced practice clinicians to order medications, diagnostic tests, and treatments independently, whereas traditional nurses require physician orders to implement these interventions (Sondergaard et al, 2024).
- Scope of Responsibility encompasses accountability for clinical outcomes, diagnostic accuracy, and treatment efficacy. This expanded responsibility reflects the autonomous nature of advanced practice and distinguishes it from the delegated authority characteristic of traditional nursing (Sondergaard et al, 2024, Schulunegger et al, 2024, Thomas et al, 2012).

Future practice

In future, although some of this is emerging now, there will be expanded surgical responsibilities assuming more of what has been traditionally viewed as physician-led practice. It is seen to a degree now, but will be seen extensively in independent surgeries, family practice, and women's health/gynecology. In addition, there will be expanded roles and responsibilities in technology, in robotics, and, overall, in the scope of responsibility for patient care delivery.

Conclusion

Advanced clinical practice represents a sophisticated evolution of nursing, and allied health positions, that extends professional boundaries and expands healthcare delivery capacity. The integration of core competencies, comprehensive scope of practice, and evidence-based approaches positions advanced practice clinicians as essential contributors to modern healthcare systems. As healthcare demands continue to evolve, advanced practice clinicians will increasingly lead innovative care models, drive quality improvement, and shape the future of patient care delivery.

References

Bales, G., Hasemann, W., Kressig, R. W., Mayer, H. (2025) Impact, scope of practice and competencies of Advanced Practice Nurses within APN-led models of care for young and middle-aged adult patients with multimorbidity and/or complex chronic conditions in hospital settings: a scoping review protocol. BMJ Open. 15(4):e091170. doi: 10.1136/bmjopen-2024-091170 https://pmc.ncbi.nlm.nih.gov/articles/PMC12039040/ (Accessed 2/24/2026).

Schlunegger, M. C., Aeschlimann, S., Palm, R., Shaha, M. Z. (2021) Competencies and scope of practice of nurse practitioners in primary health care: a scoping review protocol. www.bfh.ch/dam/jcr:0d6bdf28-1704-4345-a6ad-842b9ee87f15/Schlunegger_et_al_Competencies-Scope_of_Practice_APN_2021.pdf (Accessed 2/25/2026).

Sondergaard, S. F., Andersen, A. B., Frederiksen, K. (2024) APN nurses' core competencies for general clinical health assessment in primary health care. A scoping review. *Scandanavian Journal of Casring Science*, 38(2):258–272. https://onlinelibrary.wiley.com/doi/10.1111/scs.13235 (Accessed 2/25/2026).

Thomas, A. C., Crabtree, M. K., Delaney, K. R., Dumas, M. A., Kleinpell, R., Logsdon, C., Marfell, J., Nativio, D. (2012) Nurse Practitioner Competencies (Amended 2012) NONPF(2011) Core Competencies.pdf www.pncb.org/sites/default/files/2017-02/ (Accessed 2/24/2026).

CHAPTER 1

From the beginning to advanced practice

An expanded historical narrative

Carol L. Cox, Marie C. Hill and Victoria M. Lack

Introduction

In this chapter the history of nursing is described, both in the United Kingdom (UK) and United States of America (USA). Following this, there is a detailed discussion on how advanced nursing practice, and more recently how advanced clinical practice developed from its nursing roots, up until the present day, with a particular focus on advanced clinical practice in the UK from 2010.

Background

Nightingale's revolutionary work (1854–1860)

Florence Nightingale's contributions to nursing during the Crimean War (1854–1856) marked the beginning of modern professional nursing. Her systematic approach to patient care, environmental health, and statistical analysis revolutionized healthcare delivery. Nightingale's observations during the Crimean War led to her understanding that more soldiers died from preventable diseases than from battle wounds, prompting her to implement rigorous sanitation practices that dramatically reduced mortality rates from 42% to 2% (Bostridge, 2008).

Following her return from the Crimean War, Nightingale established the first professional nursing school at St. Thomas's Hospital in London in 1860. It was not until 1873, a watershed year, that professional nursing education began in the USA, fashioned after the Nightingale model. The Nightingale model formalized nursing education through structured curricula that emphasized both theoretical knowledge and practical skills. The Nightingale Training School became the model for nursing education worldwide by establishing principles that continue to influence contemporary nursing practice (McDonald, 2010). Nightingale's student, Ethel Gordon Bedford Fenwick, would later become instrumental in advancing nursing's professional status through regulatory frameworks.

Standards of practice and professional recognition

Ethel Gordon Bedford Fenwick emerged as a pivotal figure in establishing nursing as a legitimate profession with standardized practices. As a nurse and nurse educator, she founded the International Council of Nurses in 1899 and the British College of

DOI: 10.4324/9781003609049-2

Nurses, demonstrating remarkable leadership in professional organization development (Rafferty, 1996).

Fenwick's most significant contribution was her campaign for nationally recognized certification in nursing, which directly challenged Nightingale's more informal approach to nursing education. She argued that without proper certification and licensing, the title of 'nurse' could not be protected, leaving patients vulnerable to unqualified practitioners. This advocacy led to the establishment of standards of practice and the licensing structure that forms the foundation of contemporary nursing regulation (Abel-Smith, 1960).

Foundation of district nursing (1859)

The establishment of district nursing in 1859 established a revolutionary approach to community-based healthcare delivery which formed the foundation for public health nursing today. This approach to healthcare, initially in the home and then expanding into the community (through public health systems), provided trained nurses with specialty skills to care for patients outside the acute care/hospital setting. The initial focus of these nurses was primarily serving the poor and underserved populations who could not afford hospital care. District nursing addressed the growing recognition that health promotion and disease prevention required healthcare services to extend beyond institutional walls (Stocks, 2024).

The district nursing model emphasized holistic patient care within the community context, considering social determinants of health and family dynamics in treatment planning. As stated previously, this approach laid the groundwork for contemporary community nursing and public health nursing practices, demonstrating the profession's early commitment to health equity and accessible care (Dingwall et al., 1988).

British Nurses Association creation (1887)

The formation of the British Nurses Association (BNA) in 1887 marked a crucial step toward professional organization and collective advocacy within nursing. This association provided a formal structure and arena for nurses to collaborate on professional standards, education requirements, and working conditions. The creation of this organization served as a precursor to modern nursing unions and professional bodies, which established precedents for collective bargaining and professional representation (Abel-Smith, 1960).

Initially, the BNA work focused on elevating nursing's professional status through standardized education, ethical guidelines, and advocacy for improved working conditions. Undoubtedly, these efforts contributed to nursing's evolution from a largely unregulated occupation to a recognized healthcare profession with distinct competencies and responsibilities (Rafferty, 1996).

Formal registration through the Nurses' Acts of 1903 and 1919

In the USA, North Carolina was the first state in which formal registration became law in 1903. It enacted the Practice Act which promulgated standards for professional registration. New York, New Jersey, and Virginia followed shortly thereafter in the same year. Other states across the USA followed, elevating nursing to a respected and regulated profession (Gould, 2025.) The primary focus of regulation in the USA was and is patient safety.

In the UK, the Nurses Registration Act of 1919 represented a landmark achievement in nursing professionalization, establishing the first legal framework for nursing registration. This legislation created the General Nursing Council, which was responsible for maintaining professional standards, overseeing education, and managing the nursing register that opened in 1921 (Abel-Smith, 1960).

Following the USA, the UK Nurses' Registration Act established minimum educational requirements for nursing practice and created mechanisms for disciplinary action against practitioners who violated professional standards. This regulatory framework provided public protection while simultaneously elevating nursing's professional status through legal recognition of its specialized knowledge and skills (Dingwall et al., 1988).

Wartime contributions of nurses

Throughout both World Wars and in Korea, Vietnam, the Falklands, and the invasion of Iraq in 2003, nurses have demonstrated exceptional adaptability and clinical expertise under extreme conditions. During World War I, nurses served in field hospitals, casualty clearing stations, and hospital ships, often working in dangerous conditions close to combat zones. Their contributions extended beyond traditional patient care to include triage, emergency surgery assistance, and psychological support for traumatized soldiers (Hallett, 2009).

World War II further extended nursing roles as healthcare demands intensified on both military and civilian fronts. Nurses took on increased responsibilities in emergency medicine, trauma care, and public health initiatives. These wartime experiences accelerated the development of specialized nursing skills and demonstrated the profession's capacity for innovation and leadership in crisis situations (Brooks & Hallett, 2015). This marked the beginning of what is now termed advanced nursing practice. As wartime methods have accelerated in their development and implementation, nurses' ability to provide sophisticated care has expanded.

Establishment of the UK National Health Service (1948)

Unlike the USA, in which the provision of healthcare is reimbursed through private health insurance (i.e., Medicare and Medicaid), the creation of the National Health Service (NHS) in 1948 fundamentally converted healthcare delivery by establishing universal healthcare free at the point of service. This transformative and revolutionary system positioned nurses as essential providers within a comprehensive healthcare framework that prioritized equity and accessibility over ability to pay (Webster, 2002).

The NHS standardized education and practice across the UK; subsequently creating new opportunities for nursing specialization, career advancement, and advanced practice. Nurses became integral to the NHS success, providing continuity of care across primary, secondary, and tertiary healthcare settings. The NHS model has influenced healthcare systems globally and established principles of universal access that continue to shape contemporary healthcare policy (Klein, 2013).

Educational reforms – Project 2000 and university-based education

The Project 2000 transition in the UK culminated in 2009 when all of nursing education moved to university-based, degree-level programs. This change aligned nursing education with other healthcare professions such as medical, dental, and allied health professionals. Project 2000 provided nurses with enhanced analytical skills, research competences, and theoretical knowledge necessary for contemporary practice. This recognized nursing as an academic discipline requiring sophisticated intellectual preparation (NMC, 2010).

In the USA, nursing began matriculating from diploma to baccalaureate education in 1909 with the first Bachelor of Science in nursing at the University of Minnesota. During the 1920's and 1930's there were an increasing number of nursing programmes operating at degree level. The major change to degree-level education occurs after the Nurse Training Act of 1964. This landmark federal act heavily funded nursing education at university level. It provided major funding to develop baccalaureate, advanced (Master's), and PhD programs. This educational shift to baccalaureate and advanced degrees was strongly supported by the American Nurses Association (ANA) in the 1950s and beyond (Gurnick Academy, 2022).

It was during this period that nurse practitioner programs changed from diploma to degree and advanced practice as a discipline was establishing its foothold in healthcare provision.

United Kingdom Central Council for Nursing, Midwifery and Health Visiting (1983)

The establishment of the United Kingdom Central Council (UKCC) in 1983 created a unified regulatory framework for nursing, midwifery, and health visiting across the UK. The UKCC replaced numerous separate regulatory bodies with a single organization responsible for professional standards, education oversight, and public protection (Dingwall et al., 1988). It established a new professional register with four distinct branches: adult nursing, children's nursing, mental health nursing, and learning disability nursing. This structure recognized the specialized knowledge and skills required for different patient populations while maintaining common professional standards across all nursing specialties (Dingwall et al., 1988).

Founding of the Nursing and Midwifery Council (2002)

The Nursing and Midwifery Council (NMC), established in 2002, replaced the UKCC as the regulatory body for nursing and midwifery in the UK. The NMC's creation reflected evolving healthcare needs and the profession's growing autonomy and responsibility. This organization maintains professional registers, sets education standards, and provides guidance on professional conduct (NMC, 2002).

The NMC's regulatory framework emphasizes public protection through rigorous standards for professional competence, continuing education requirements, and accountability mechanisms. The organization's work ensures that nurses and midwives maintain current knowledge and skills throughout their careers while upholding ethical standards that protect patient safety and welfare (NMC, 2018). Presently the NMC is studying regulation of Advanced Nursing Practice as it is regulated at national and state level in the USA.

Advanced Practice Nursing, as it is known in the USA, started developing in the USA in the early 1940s with the establishment of Nurse Anaesthetists and Nurse Midwives. The first Nurse Practitioner Program was established in 1965 by Dr. Lorette Ford and Dr. Henry Silver at the University of Colorado, leading to state regulation in the 1970s and National Consistency with the 2008 Advanced Practice Registered Nurse (APRN) Consensus Model for standardized licensure and certification. The 2008 Consensus Model was released by the National Council of State Boards of Nursing (NCSBN) and the American Association of Colleges of Nursing (AACN). It guided all states toward uniform regulation, licensure, accreditation, and certification. Advanced Practice spans disciplines including Advanced Practice Registered Nurses (APRNs), Certified Registered Nurse Anaesthetists, Certified Nurse Midwives, and Clinical Nurse Specialists. APRNs specialize, for example, in family practice, pediatrics, women's health, obstetrics and gynecology, or mental health. In most states, APRNs have full practice authority, including prescribing and independent practice. However, according to the American Association of Nurse Practitioners (AANP) challenges are present as state laws are varied with some states limiting full formulary prescribing (AANP, 2025).

In the UK prescribing rights were granted to nurses practicing at an advanced level in 2002, following completion of a prescribing course as part of the advanced practice program. Prior to this time, the prescribing qualification had to be completed at a different time to the program. The extension of prescribing rights to appropriately qualified nurses in 2002 marked a significant expansion of nursing's scope of practice.

This development recognized nurses' clinical expertise and their capacity to make independent therapeutic decisions within their areas of competence. Nurse prescribing initially focused on specific conditions and medications but gradually expanded to include a broader range of therapeutic interventions (Latter & Courtenay, 2004).

As noted above, this advancement required additional education and assessment of competencies to ensure patient safety while providing nurses with greater autonomy in patient care. Prescribing rights enhanced care continuity and efficiency while demonstrating nursing's evolution toward advanced practice roles that complement and extend traditional medical practice (Courtenay et al., 2007). It is worthy of note that this educational advancement positioned nursing alongside other healthcare professions requiring university-level preparation and contributed to improved patient outcomes through enhanced clinical decision-making capabilities. The degree requirement has also facilitated nursing's continued evolution toward advanced practice roles and leadership positions within healthcare systems in the UK (Health Education England and NMC, 2015).

Advent of independent nursing research

Nursing research is recognized as having its beginnings with the work undertaken by Florence Nightengale. Its evolution has been gradual. In the mid 20th century, nursing research focused on patient outcomes, nursing theories, and educational methods. Although nursing research was formalized in the USA in the 1960s with university education (Gurnick Academy of Medical Arts, 2022), the formal recognition of independent nursing research in the UK came to the fore in 2010. With this recognition nursing became established as a distinct academic discipline capable of generating knowledge that informs practice and policy. This development acknowledged nursing's unique perspective on health, illness, and healthcare delivery while providing mechanisms for systematic inquiry into nursing-specific phenomena (Gurnick Academy of Medical Arts, 2022).

Independent research capacity enables nurses to investigate questions most relevant to nursing practice, develop nursing-specific interventions, and contribute to interdisciplinary healthcare knowledge. This research foundation supports evidence-based practice and provides the scientific basis for nursing's continued evolution toward advanced practice roles with expanded scope and autonomy (Flanagan and Beck, 2024).

Advanced practice in the USA is eloquently described by Jane Sumner in this book. Therefore, additional discussion regarding advanced practice in the USA will not focus further in this chapter. Rather the focus shifts to the important work that has been and is being undertaken in the UK, beginning with the Council for Regulatory Healthcare Regulatory Excellence report (CHRE, 2009) and the Department of Health's position statement on advanced-level practice in 2010 (DoH, 2010).

Council for Healthcare Regulatory Excellence (2009), and UK Department of Health (2010) position statement on advanced-level practice

Since its inception in the late 1980s in the UK, advanced practice in healthcare has suffered from a lack of clarity and recognition. Whereas the nurse practitioner in the USA is recognized by public and professionals as an individual that is a competent clinician with postgraduate training and who has passed a national examination enabling them to practice independently, in the UK there is not such understanding or recognition.

In 2008, after many years of debate about definitions, educational preparation, and regulation, the Council for Healthcare Regulatory Excellence (CHRE) was asked by the Secretary of State for Health in the UK to examine advanced practice and to consider the necessity for regulation. The rationale for undertaking the review was to ensure that patient and public safety was not being put at risk because of advanced practice. The CHRE published its report in 2009 (CHRE, 2009). It found that there had been inconsistency in how the term 'advanced practice' had been applied to different healthcare professionals' roles. It indicated that this had frequently led to confusion about the scope and competence required at an advanced level of practice and confirmed the need for a set of nationally agreed standards for advanced-level practice to support employers and commissioners in order to ensure good governance arrangements (CHRE, 2009; DoH, 2010). However, the report concluded that advanced practice was not a regulatory issue, and highlighted that:

> *Risks to patient safety come from professionals taking on roles and responsibilities for which they are not competent to carry out safely and effectively, or because of inadequate safeguards.*
>
> *Employers are responsible for assessing fitness for purpose of their employees and job applicants with regard to the competencies (competence) required for the given job. Employers are in a position to determine this by considering the specific roles and responsibilities the professional would be taking on.*
>
> *Employers and commissioners need to ensure that robust organisational governance is in place to manage risks to patient safety from individuals in relation to*

competence and safeguards and that self-employed professionals are under a duty of care not to practise in ways in which they are not competent to do safely and to ensure that in the service they provide the necessary steps are taken to ensure patients are not put at unwarranted risk of harm and also that they keep their skills current in relation to their scope of practice.

(CHRE, 2009; Refer specifically to pp. 11–13)

The CHRE report therefore concluded that the primary issues associated with patient safety related to practitioners not being competent and/or employers not providing safeguards. It stated that a workforce that periodically demonstrates fitness for practice (for example through revalidation) should be up-to-date and fit for purpose. Although the view of the CHRE was that the regulation of advanced practice was not necessary, it was clear that standards for advanced practice were required. 'It is the core role of the regulatory body to assure a professional's fitness to practise the profession, through setting and enforcing standards of proficiency and conduct' (CHRE, 2009: p6). The CHRE report laid the burden of competence firmly with the employer to enforce. Unfortunately, employers did not do this, but added to the confusion by introducing a plethora of titles for nurses, and other practitioners, with varying skills and abilities. This led to continued and further misunderstanding among health professionals, not to mention the general public, about what exactly a nurse practitioner or advanced clinical practitioner is or can do.

In October 2017 the combined Professional Bodies and Royal Colleges representing the health workforce in the UK produced a joint professional statement, committing to work together in the interests of the health of the nation, through promotion of the strengths of different professions within teams. The result was the "Multi-Professional Framework for Advanced Clinical Practice in England" (HEE, 2017). It set out a *new and bold vision in developing this critical workforce role (i.e. Advanced Clinical Practitioners (ACPs) in a consistent way to ensure safety, quality and effectiveness* (p4). The purpose of this framework was to build on the work already done in the four nations in the UK (i.e., England, Wales, Scotland, and Northern Ireland) and to enable a consistent understanding of what advanced clinical practice is. For the first time this framework gives one definition of advanced clinical practice to which all key stakeholders have agreed, and a list of 'capabilities' that all ACPs must have. This is important, as until then, different professions and Royal Colleges had different definitions and different ideas about the skills and knowledge that ACPs should have. It is important to note, however, that the framework applies only to England.

The agreed definition of advanced clinical practice was:

Advanced clinical practice is delivered by experienced, registered health and care practitioners. It is a level of practice characterised by a high degree of autonomy and complex decision making. This is underpinned by a master's level award or equivalent that encompasses the four pillars of clinical practice, leadership and management, education and research, with demonstration of core capabilities and area specific clinical competence. Advanced clinical practice embodies the ability to manage clinical care in partnership with individuals, families and carers. It includes the analysis and synthesis of complex problems across a range of settings, enabling innovative solutions to enhance people's experience and improve outcomes.

The framework further states that:

> *This definition therefore requires that health and care professionals working at the level of advanced clinical practice will exercise autonomy and decision making in a context of complexity, uncertainty and varying levels of risk, holding accountability for decisions made.*
>
> (HEE, 2017: p8)

In this agreed definition, autonomy, decision-making, and complexity are reinforced. The preparation of clinicians, which had been long debated, is clarified as requiring a Master's-level award, although it withdraws from saying this is essential. It also breaks down advanced clinical practice into four 'pillars' which then form the basis for grouping the knowledge and skills necessary, which the framework calls 'capabilities.' These four pillars are different from the DOH 2010 position statement and are partly based on evidence from an action research study which put into practice the advanced practice/consultant nurse role in a Nursing Development Unit in London (Manley, 1997). The final, perhaps more subtle, point is that the ACP is expected to demonstrate these core capabilities and 'area'-specific competence. This is a nod to the increasing diversity of advanced clinical practice over the proceeding few years and allows for different professional groups and specialisms within those professions to define themselves as ACPs.

The four pillars of advanced clinical practice were (HEE, 2017):

(1) Clinical practice
(2) Leadership and management
(3) Education
(4) Research

In the years following the Multi-Professional Framework, much has been made of the fact that ACPs need to demonstrate capability in all four areas. Whilst acknowledging that not all ACPs will practice equally in all four areas, the framework makes exceptionally high demands on ACPs that they can work to 'master's level' in these four pillars of practice. This framework also considers workforce planning and enabling ACPs to be placed in roles in which they will be able to use their skill to make a difference. It also discusses the educational preparation of ACPs.

Education for advance practice

Prior to the Multi-Professional Framework (HEE, 2017), there were no enforced standards for the preparation of ACPs. To fill this gap, the Royal College of Nursing (RCN) had devised a system of accreditation of ACP programs. Higher Educational Institutions (HEIs) could become accredited RCN courses by demonstrating adherence to the RCN guidelines and by payment of a fee. This was desirable for HEI's as it could help to attract students, as there was the suggestion that if advanced clinical practice was regulated in the future, then the RCN-accredited courses would fulfill the criteria for educational preparation. In 2016 Health Education England (HEE) set out Standards for Education and Training, which defined what a Master's-level Advanced Clinical Practice program should look like. In order to gain accreditation, the programme had to already be in existence; to be validated by the individual HEI; to map against the capabilities of the Multi-Professional Framework and the Standards for Education and Training of the HEI (NHS England, n.d.). In addition, the ACP program must demonstrate a person-centered and a learner-centered approach, demonstrate learning in the workplace, and have the following program content (NHS England, n.d.):

- Facilitate and develop Advanced Practice-level learning across all the pillars of practice
- Integrate and blend learning to optimize experience and outcomes (within academic and learning in practice settings)
- Promote professionalism and consideration of ethical issues and personal scope of practice and competence (and their limits)
- Place a strong emphasis on
  - Self-directed learning
  - Accountability and responsibility for personal decisions and actions
  - Collaborative practice
  - Reflection on the management of complexity, uncertainty, and ethical issues
  - Critical inquiry and evidence-based practice
  - High level of autonomy
  - Clinical decision-making
  - Exercising of informed judgment

Initially, HEIs had to apply to HEE for accreditation. A Centre for Advancing Practice was then established which took over this role. On completion of an accredited program, ACPs were eligible to apply for a 'digital badge' which would demonstrate to employers (and the public) that they had graduated from a program recognized by HEE, or more recently from the Centre for Advancing Practice. As of August 2025, 59 universities have this accreditation for their ACP programs (NHS England, 2025a). In addition to the credentialing of programs, the Centre for Advancing Practice also offers a route to obtaining the digital badge via a professional portfolio. This involves registering with an approved HEI and completion of a portfolio demonstrating advanced practice capabilities, which can then lead to the 'digital badge.'

Funding for advanced practice courses initially relied on self-funding by practitioners themselves, interested NHS trusts, and/or 'good will' of General Practices. In the 2010s funding was available from HEE (in England) for tuition fees and for 'backfill' to cover the ACP while in training. However, the amount of support available differed across the country. Following this, the possibility of undertaking MSc ACP programs using a government-funded apprenticeship levy arose in the 2010s and has subsequently been taken up by many HEIs. This is a system whereby the student is supported by the employer to undertake an MSc ACP program which is tailored to fulfill the requirements of an apprenticeship program. Apprenticeship programs include additional requirements in terms of workplace meetings and supervision and must also include an 'End Pont Assessment' (EPA) where the student ACP must demonstrate competency in all four pillars through an exam and presentation of practice (Skills England, n.d.). The EPA is strictly regulated and involves an Independent Assessor (an ACP who is also experienced in academic assessments, who is independent of the HEI) as well as an Internal Moderator, who is from the HEI but is not involved in the ACP program.

The student is marked against an extensive rubric, involving essential criteria in all four pillars which must be passed. This is in addition to fulfilling all the requirements of the remainder of the ACP program.

For the first time then, for apprenticeship students at least, there is to some extent a national program of assessment, although there is no mandated moderation between HEIs. However, the Association of Advanced Practice Educators (AAPE) were given the task to establish a national framework for assessment and marking to promote consistency across England. Again, the apprenticeship system does not apply to the other three countries of the UK. Feedback from students and HEIs is mixed regarding the assessment: it can feel like students are assessed twice (once through the HEI program and then again through the EPA). In addition, the wording of the rubrics is complex in places, and therefore to answer questions demonstrating competency in all areas of practice is challenging for teachers to teach, and students to achieve. Apprenticeships at level 7 have mostly been abandoned by the government in 2025. However, ACP apprenticeships have been given a reprieve for now, presumably due to the demand for ACPs in the workplace.

Advanced practice in primary care

In 2020, HEE, The Royal College of General Practitioners (RCGPs), and Skills for Health issued a document; "Core Capabilities framework for Advanced Clinical Practice (Nurses) Working in General Practice/Primary Care in England" (HEE et al., 2020). The purpose of this framework was to set out the standard and to "give practitioners the opportunity to develop and evidence their knowledge and skills, enabling highest standards of practice, as well as providing a structure for career and role development within primary care" (HEE et al., 2020: p5). Again, this document applies to England only and specifically to nurses. It acknowledges the Multi-Professional Framework (HEE, 2017), but divides 'capabilities' into four domains rather than four pillars as in Table 1.1 below:

Table 1.1 gives more emphasis to the clinical element of practice than the Multi-Professional Framework and highlights the importance of clinical skills and condition management. This Core Clinical Capabilities for Advanced Clinical Practice (Nurses) (HEE et al., 2020) framework is intended as a guide for service commissioners,

Table 1.1 Pillars of the ACP Framework

Pillars of the ACP Framework	*Domains of the Core Capabilities Framework for Advanced Clinical Practitioners (Nurses) Working in General Practice/Primary Care*
1. Clinical Practice	Domain A. Person-centered collaborative working Domain B. Assessment, investigations, and diagnosis Domain C. Condition management, treatment, and prevention
2. Leadership and Management **3. Education** **4. Research**	Domain D. Leadership and management, education, and research

Source: HEE et al. (2020: p12).

employers, HEIs, clinical supervisors, and ACPs in Primary Care, to understand the minimum standards required to fulfill the role in the Primary Care setting and to be able to demonstrate capability. There is a portfolio for students to complete so they can demonstrate their competency as ACPs in Primary Care. In my experience in using this portfolio within a MSc ACP program, it is a robust and comprehensive way to ensure that a wide range of advanced practice knowledge and skills in Primary Care are evidenced; albeit that it is a lengthy task to undertake. It is interesting however that HEE were fundamental to the development of both the Multi-Professional Framework (HEE, 2017) and The Core Clinical Capabilities for Advanced Clinical Practice (Nurses) (HEE et al., 2020) but have allowed such differences to exist, such as the four pillars in the Multi-Professional Framework (HEE, 2017) and the four domains of practice in The Core Clinical Capabilities for Advanced Clinical Practice (Nurses) (HEE et al., 2020).

Other areas of advanced practice

With the increasing diversity of practitioners becoming interested in achieving 'advanced practice status,' HEE, and subsequently the newly created Centre for Advancing Practice, have developed and endorsed more specialist areas of practice; thereby re-opening an old debate around the difference between specialist and advanced practice. Areas that now have area-specific competencies attached, which can be 'endorsed' by the Centre for Advancing Practice include (Centre for Advancing Practice, n.d.):

(Acute Cardiology)
Autism
Community-based rehabilitation: physical activity for people with long-term conditions
Learning disability
Musculo-skeletal conditions
(Non-surgical oncology)
Pelvic Health
Public Health
(Sexual Health/HIV)
Acute medicine
Community-based rehabilitation: health ageing
End-of-life care
Mental Health
Neurological rehabilitation
Older People
Pediatric and Child Health
Respiratory
(Surgery)

The areas of practice in brackets are still in the process of gaining endorsement by the Centre for Advancing Practice, the remainder were endorsed in the early 2020s. If this looks like a rather random selection of areas of practice; some with a very large scope of practice, such as acute medicine, and some with a very specific scope, such as pelvic health, that is because it probably is. The development of these specialist areas has been very much led by practitioners themselves, rather than by a combined effort to cover areas where ACPs are needed and require area-specific skills. The idea is, however, that ACPs gain their generic ACP qualification and later (or possibly at the same time) develop more specific skills.

In addition, different Royal Colleges, such as the RCGP, have devised their own competencies for development of advanced practice in certain areas. For example, the Royal College of Emergency Medicine (RCEM) since 2015 have developed a curriculum and credentialing process for Emergency Care ACPs to provide a consistent standard in education and training for ACPs in Emergency Departments. The process is now a standard part of RCEM activity (RCEM, n.d.). The RCEM response to the lack of regulation and protection of the ACP title, and lack of consistency in the abilities of ACPs has led to a robust framework of Emergency Department (ED) ACP practice, which has enabled ACPs working in this area to develop robust and consistent skills across the UK.

The NMC

The corporate strategy of the NMC 2020–2025 committed to undertaking a comprehensive review of Advanced Practice across the UK. This was largely based on work commissioned by the NMC and undertaken by the Nuffield Trust (Palmer et al, 2023). This review found that nurses, and to a lesser extent midwives, are increasingly taking on *more complex, autonomous and expert roles commonly referred to as 'advanced practice'* (Palmer et al, 2023: p4). In addition, the review notes that there is currently no specific additional regulation covering advanced practice, and as a result nurses and midwives themselves are responsible for ensuring they work within existing regulatory frameworks and employers are responsible for ensuring that nurses (and midwives) are suitably qualified and experienced for any advanced practice role. Palmer et al. noted that 11 countries outside the UK have nurses working at a similar level of advanced practice to nurses in the UK, but only Finland (alongside the four nations of the UK) does not regulate advanced practice (Palmer et al., 2023). Only one country (Republic of Ireland) specifically regulates advanced midwifery practice. The authors further elaborated that there are risks with current arrangements, although evidence is limited as this is a small (but growing) group of professionals in the UK (Palmer et al., 2023). Participants in research carried out by Palmer et al. (2023) found there was an increased risk of harm to people using advanced practice services, particularly where the employer was not an NHS organization. Some participants in the research have suggested that this particularly applies to General Practice (GP) and Out Of Hours (OOH) services, nursing homes, and agencies. The authors also reported that there was poor understanding by the public of what advanced practice is, which could undermine consent to treatment.

The Report (Palmer et al., 2023) found a considerable variation in preparation for nurses and midwives in advanced practice, which is of concern. This is different from Australia, New Zealand, and the USA, where ACP regulation means that there are national stands that have to be attained. There was also concern that while it is appropriate to have a degree of difference to approaches to advanced practice across the four nations of the UK, there is a risk if they become too divergent, especially if clinicians move to work in other regions of the UK. Overall, 78% of stakeholders from other clinical professions were in favor of specific regulation of advanced practice (Hardy, 2021, cited by Palmer et al., 2023). The full report makes interesting reading, and explores the complexity of regulating advanced practice, and the different ways that it could be done (Palmer et al., 2023). However, the result of the report is in favor of regulation, but that it needs to be carefully thought out, considered in the context of providing clarity on the protection of the 'nurse' title, and should apply to all four nations of the UK.

In July 2023, as part of the NMC review, the NMC also commissioned qualitative research into Advanced Practice by 'Britain Thinks' (2023). Forty-nine nurses and 15 midwives from across the four nations in the UK took part in focus groups and in-depth interviews. The sample size was small, compared to the number of nurses and midwives in the UK, but there are conclusions from this that are worth noting. The research confirmed the great variation in scope and use of advanced practice roles, and some flexibility to meet the demands of the employer and people they care for is good. However, with this is also risk; there is a high degree of variation in preparation for advanced practice across the four nations which can lead to a variation in the level of skills of professionals. This can lead to mixed expectations of employers and a degree of mistrust from members of the public. It can also lead to professionals working beyond their scope of practice, and the lack of boundaries is risky to the ACPs themselves as there is no clear protection. In summary the research found that there are factors which are common to most advanced practice roles (autonomy, complex decision-making, and treating complex cases). In the case of midwives, who are autonomous at registration, the defining factor is complexity. Outside of this, the roles of ACPs are heterogenous. The professionals interviewed in this qualitative research considered that ACPs provide benefit to patients, especially in providing continuity of care, as opposed to, for example, rotating medical staff. However, the heterogeneity of advanced practice means that neither the advanced practice nurses/midwives nor the general public knew exactly what to expect of an advanced practitioner and therefore, overall, the professional felt that regulation, introduced carefully, would be supportive of their role.

Using evidence from the above two reports as well as other evidence, the NMC advised their council in 2023 to engage a steering group to advise on next steps. This resulted in the development of a set of advanced practice principles, to be followed by the development of standards of proficiency and associated advanced practice program standards at a later date. This will include more public consultation. Phase three will then be about transition and implementation of standards (NMC 2025a). In June 2025, the NMC announced a new definition and principles for advanced practice (NMC, 2025b). The definition seeks to bring consistency for all nurses and midwives, both clinical and non-clinical, working at an advanced practice level. There are two versions:

The professional version

A Registered Nurse or Midwife working at an advance level is an expert professional working with additional postgraduate education and experience. They use their education-informed knowledge, skills, and capability to influence, shape, deliver, and lead safe and effective care, while managing risk, uncertainty, and complexity.

The public version

A Registered Nurse or Midwife working at an advance level of practice is a professional who has completed extra post-qualification education to increase their knowledge and skills, allowing them to deliver and lead expert, higher-level care (NMC, 2025c: p8).

There are 12 principles for individual professionals, see Box 1.1:

Box 1.1 Principles of Advanced Practice*

These principles provide clear expectations for advanced-level practice across a range of roles and settings. These roles can span wide areas of health and social care aligned to local and national legal, regulatory, professional, and educational requirements. This includes but is not limited to the delivery of safe and effective care for a range of people across the continuum of care with a well-developed understanding of the wider determinants of health to safeguard and promote wellbeing, protect health, and prevent ill health.

All nurses and midwives on our register must practice in line with the Code. In addition, advanced-level practitioners should:

1.1 Practice within their individual scope of practice and in line with their level of knowledge, experience, qualifications, training, and employment role.
1.2 Demonstrate expertise, confidence, critical thinking, and evidence appraisal and synthesis within their individual scope of practice to lead and influence education, research, and practice.
1.3 Demonstrate professional accountability and capability in making complex evidence-informed decisions, managing varying degrees of risk, unpredictability, and uncertainty while exercising professional judgment. This includes using initiative, demonstrating significant autonomy, and being accountable for their actions.
1.4 Demonstrate self-awareness with compassionate and inspirational leadership within inter-professional teams to influence practice for effective, holistic, person-centered care.
1.5 Demonstrate use of evidence-informed expert knowledge to practice reflectively, identifying areas for self-improvement and improved outcomes for a diverse range of individuals, teams, and people.
1.6 Role model reflective and reflexive practice and advocate for access to individualized support and clinical supervision to ensure continuous learning, improvement, and professional development across the four pillars.
1.7 Role model professional practice, advocating for and contributing to inter-professional learning and working to provide leadership and effective support and supervision to a broad range of colleagues and learners.
1.8 Use their expert, advanced-level knowledge and experience to challenge themselves and others to promote and embed professional curiosity and the principles of equality, equity, diversity, and inclusion in their area of practice, seeking and acting upon feedback received from peers, colleagues, and the public.
1.9 Support, influence, and lead projects in the environments they work in to shape a reflective learning culture where safety, quality, continuous improvement, and sustainability are prioritized, including promoting allyship and advocacy for all, speaking up and raising concerns where required.
1.10 Evidence continued capability, reflective and reflexive practice, ongoing learning, and professional development at an advanced level, relevant to their scope of practice through local appraisal processes and through professional revalidation requirements.

1.11 Utilize their expertise and experience to minimise environmental impacts, enhance economic growth, and embed sustainable approaches to service planning, delivery, and implementation.
1.12 Lead and contribute to the proactive identification and resolution of challenges to health, safety, and wellbeing for individuals and population groups, shaping the design and delivery of effective services and policies that promote holistic health and wellbeing.

Note: *NMC (2025b: pp 14–15).

There are also principles for employing organizations to ensure, for example, governance processes are addressed and that there is a culture that supports ongoing learning opportunities.

It is interesting that the NMC has moved from a position in 2010, in which advanced practice was not seen as something which needed additional regulation, to the current position, in which the NMC has taken the evidence on board that regulation is what nurses, midwives, and other health professionals actually want. It is unclear whether these definitions, which are broad so as to encompass all possible areas of 'advanced practice,' will actually help professionals and the public to understand what Advanced Practitioners actually do, and if they will be robust enough to protect the public. Hopefully more clarity will emerge as the principles are developed into standards of proficiency.

At the same time as the NMC have been developing their definition and principles, the Centre for Advancing Practice has issued an update of the Multi-Professional Framework for Advanced Practice in England. (NHS England, 2025b).

The first thing to notice is that the word 'clinical' has been removed from the title: This is because, the Centre for Advancing Practice state, the use of the word clinical gave the impression that advanced practice is a generic role, as opposed to a level of practice which encompasses areas of practice where the word 'clinical' feels "less relevant" (NHS England, 2025b: p12).

The definition of advanced practice as agreed by all stakeholders is:

> Advanced practice is delivered by accomplished registered health and care professionals. It is a level of practice characterised by a high degree of autonomy and designated responsibility for complex decision making. This is underpinned by a post-registration master's level award or equivalent undertaken by an experienced practitioner that encompasses all four pillars of clinical practice, leadership and management, education, and research. Advanced practice embodies the ability to manage care in partnership with individuals, families, and carers. It includes the analysis and synthesis of complex problems, and management of clinical risk and uncertainty across a range of settings, enabling innovative solutions to expedite access to care, optimise people's experiences, and improve outcomes.
>
> (NHS England, 2025a: p5)

There are a few subtle differences between the 2017 version and the 2025 definition: as stated, the word 'clinical' has been taken out (it occurred three times in the 2017 version). Also, 'accomplished' replaces the word 'experienced', and there are a few additions to the 2025 version. The removal of the word 'clinical' indicates a move away from the original purpose of advanced practitioners, to a more heterogenous purpose which includes education, housing, and justice, according to the Multi-Professional Framework. However, the four pillars remain the same, including the clinical one. The scope of the Multidisciplinary Framework applies mainly to professions within the nine health and care professional bodies that are regulated in England and overseen by the Professional Standards Authority for Health and Social Care (PSA). It also applies only to England. However, NHS England state as part of the update in the Multi-Professional Framework that they considered the equivalent frameworks in Wales, Scotland, and Northern Ireland to ensure alignment.

Developments in Scotland, Wales, and Northern Ireland.

Scotland

There are some differences in the understanding and implementation of advanced clinical practice across the UK, especially in Scotland. The NHS Advanced Practice Toolkit is a resource for anyone working in advanced practice, whether as a practitioner, manager, or educator. It was developed in 2008 as a Scottish education resource and was endorsed UK wide by all four chief nursing officers (NHS Scotland n.d.).

The four pillars of advanced practice are used, with slight changes in nomenclature:

- Clinical Practice – knowledge, skills, and behaviors needed to provide high-quality healthcare that is safe, effective, and person-centered.
- Facilitating Learning – knowledge, skills, and behaviors needed to enable effective learning in the workplace.
- Leadership – knowledge, skills, and behaviors needed to lead and to fulfill management responsibilities.
- Evidence, Research, and Development – knowledge, skills, and behaviors needed to use evidence to inform practice and improve services.

In 2017, the Scottish Government issued a paper: "Transforming Nursing, Midwifery and Health Professions Roles: Advanced Nursing Practice" (Scottish Government, 2017). This focused on nursing roles and gave the following definition of advanced nurse practitioner:

> Advanced nurse practitioners (ANPs) are experienced and highly educated registered nurses who manage the complete clinical care of their patients, not focusing on any sole condition.

The focus was therefore on nurses, rather than other allied health practitioners, and stated that ANPs are educated at Masters level and should be operating at a minimum of agenda for change band 7. A list of ANP competencies were developed, which were clinical assessment, differential diagnosis, investigations, treatment and admission, discharge, and referral. The definition and competencies outlined in the paper are clear and easy for professionals and the public to understand and take a more 'traditional' focus than England, where the Multi-Professional Framework perhaps loses its way in trying to be all things to all people (Scottish Government, 2017). In 2021, a follow up paper was published: "Advancing Nursing Practice: Transforming Nursing Roles: Phase Two" (Scottish Government, 2021). This was intended to be an addendum to the 2017 paper. However, the competencies have been expanded to different areas of advanced practice where it was felt that more specific direction was needed: these are

- Adult Acute Care
- Pediatric Acute Care
- Neonatal Acute Care
- Adult and Pediatric Mental Health
- Adult and Pediatric Community Care

This differs from the direction taken in England where the capabilities cover all aspects of advanced practice. Although the advanced practice toolkit covers all professionals working in advanced practice, Scotland has tended to focus on ANPs rather than ACPs, although this has changed somewhat in recent years. In November 2025, the launch of Transforming Roles: Allied Health Professions Advanced Practice has been launched with the aim of setting out a vision for AHP Advanced Practice. In November 2025, Transforming roles paper 9 was launched around Allied Health professions, to set out a "national vision for AHP advanced practice" (Scottish Government, 2025).

Wales

The Professional Framework for Enhanced, Advanced and Consultant Clinical Practice (Health Education and Improvement, 2023) establishes the definition and scope of advanced practice in Wales. Key differences with the Multidisciplinary Framework for England are that extended, advanced, and consultant roles are defined. The definition of advanced practice in Wales is unchanged since 2010, being:

> *A role, requiring a registered practitioner to have acquired an expert knowledge base, complex decision-making skills, and clinical competencies for expanded scope of practice, the characteristics of which are shaped by the context in which the individual practices. Demonstrable, relevant Masters level education is recommended for entry level.*
>
> (HEIW, 2023: p25)

The Welsh framework recognizes there are practitioners who may not be working in a clinical role, and the framework will also apply to these practitioners, albeit the definition is largely clinical (Health Education and Improvement, 2023). The four pillars are the same as in the other nations.

Northern Ireland

In Northern Ireland, the Advanced AHP Practice Framework was published in 2019 (Department of Health, 2019). The definition of an Advanced Practitioner is adapted from the National Leadership and Innovation Agency 2010 and the NHS England definition from 2015. The definition of advanced practice in Northern Ireland is:

> *A role, requiring a registered experienced practitioner to have acquired an expert knowledge base, complex decision-making skills and clinical competences for expanded/extended scope of practice, the characteristics of which are shaped by the context in which the individual practices. Demonstrable, relevant education is recommended for entry level to the advanced practice role which is to be at master's level or equivalent and which meets the education, training and Continuous Professional Development (CPD) requirements for ACP as identified within the framework.*
>
> (Department of Health, 2019: p20)

The framework highlights the difference between an advanced and specialist practitioner, and again states that the Advanced Practitioner (AP) would normally be working at level 7 or above. The four pillars remain the same (Department of Health, 2019: p20).

Conclusion

This chapter focused on a brief history of nursing beginning with the era of Florence Nightingale and her groundbreaking work in the development of nursing practice. Standards of practice have been discussed which addressed the evolution of standards from basic nursing to advanced practice in the UK and the USA. The chapter then introduced the aspiring and established advanced-level nurse, midwife, and allied health professional in the UK to the most recent perspectives regarding advanced practice. It has delineated elements, domains, and competencies that are integral to the role of advanced-level practice.

Whereas in the USA, advance practice remains largely associated with advanced nursing practice, in the UK, advanced (clinical) practice has evolved from a largely nurse-based profession, to encompass a wide range of practitioners in the last 15 years. The Multi-Professional Framework in England has served to define advanced practice more clearly in England at least and may have helped to clarify the identity of an ACP/AP, as well as standardizing the level and content of educational preparation. However, even in England, the primary care framework does not tally with the Multi-Professional Framework and the different countries, especially Scotland, have different ways of defining advanced practice. The NMC have belatedly come back to the party to discuss regulation across the UK, but only for nurses. It appears today that the majority of practitioners and employers would welcome regulation. However, the remit of advanced practice is now so wide in the UK that perhaps it is impossible to provide a meaningful definition of all that is considered advanced practice.

In the chapters that follow, various concepts associated with clinical skills, management, leadership, and the professional role in advanced-level practice are explicated. Specific activities are embedded in these chapters. These activities are designed for your personal reflection and development.

References

AANP (2025). "Issues at a Glance: Full Practice Authority". American Association of Nurse Practitioners, September.

Abel-Smith, B. (1960). *A History of the Nursing Profession*. Heinemann.

Bostridge, M. (2008). *Florence Nightingale: The Making of an Icon*. Farrar, Straus and Giroux.

Britainthinks, (2023). Advanced Practice qualitative research. Available from: www.nmc.org.uk/globalassets/sitedocuments/advanced-practice-review/nmc_bt-advanced-practice_report.pdf (Accessed 24/11/25).

Brooks, J., & Hallett, C. (2015). One hundred years of nursing wartime practices, 1854–1953. *International History of Nursing Journal*, 2(1), 4–17.

Centre for Advancing Practice (n.d.). Centre-endorsed area specific frameworks. Available from Centre-endorsed area specific frameworks – Advanced Practice (Accessed 24/11/2025).

Council for Healthcare Regulatory Excellence (2009). *Advanced Practice: Report to the Four UK Health Departments. Unique ID 17–2008*. Available from: www.chre.org.uk/_img/pics/library/090709_Advanced_Practice_report_FINAL.pdf (Accessed 24/11/2025).

Courtenay, M., Carey, N., & Burke, J. (2007). Independent extended supplementary nurse prescribing practice in the UK: A national questionnaire survey. *International Journal of Nursing Studies*, 44(7), 1093–1101.

Department of Health (2010). *Advanced Level Nursing: A Position Statement*. www.dh.gov.uk/prod_consum_dh/groups/dh_digitalassets/@dh/@en/@ps/documents/digitalasset/dh_121738.pdf (Accessed 14/06/2011).

Department of Health (2019). *Advanced AHP Practice Framework*. Department of Health (Northern Ireland).

Dingwall, R., Rafferty, A. M., & Webster, C. (1988). *An Introduction to the Social History of Nursing*. London: Routledge.

Flanagan, J.M. and Beck, C.T. (2024). Generating and Assessing Evidence for Nursing Research: Twelfth International Edition. Wolters Kluwer.

Gould, D. (2025) *The Inside Story of the Nursing Profession* (1st edn). London: Routledge.

Gurnick Academy of Medical Arts (2022). "Nursing Education in the Information Age and the MSN". Available from: www.gurnick.edu/nursing-education-in-the-information-age-and-the-msn/ (Accessed 07/01/2025).

Hallett, C. (2009). *Containing Trauma: Nursing Work in the First World War*. Manchester University Press.

Hardy, M. (2021). Advanced Practice: Research report. University of Bradford. www.hcpc-uk.org/globalassets/resources/policy/independent-research-report-advanced-practice-27th-january-2021.pdf?v=637483937140000000 (Accessed 27/04/2023). IN

Health Education and Improvement Wales (2023). *Professional Framework for Enhanced, Advanced and Consultant Clinical Practice in Wales*. HEIW.

Health Education England (2017). *Multi-Professional Framework for Advanced Clinical Practice in England*. London: Health Education England.

Health Education England, NHS England and Skills for Health (2020). *Core Capabilities framework for Advanced Clinical Practice (Nurses) Working in General Practice/Primary Care in England*. London: NHS England.

Health Education England and NMC (2015). Raising the Bar. NMC.

Klein, R. (2013). *The New Politics of the NHS: From Creation to Reinvention* (7th edn). Radcliffe Publishing.

Latter, S., & Courtenay, M. (2004). Effectiveness of nurse prescribing: A review of the literature. Journal of Clinical Nursing, 13(1), 26–32.

Manley, K. (1997). A conceptual framework for advanced practice: an action research project operationalizing an advanced practitioner/consultant nurse role. *Journal of Clinical Nursing*, 6(3), 179–190.

Mcdonald, L. (Ed.). (2010). *Florence Nightingale: The Nightingale School.* Wilfrid Laurier University Press.

NHS England (n.d.). *Standards for Education and Training V2.1.* Available from: https://advanced-practice.hee.nhs.uk/standards-for-education-and-training/ (Accessed 24/11/2025).

NHS England (2025a) Accredited Programmes. Available from Accredited Programmes – Advanced Practice (Accessed 24/11/2025).

NHS England (2025b) *Multi-Professional Framework for Advanced Practice in England*: The Centre for Advancing Practice. London: NHS England.

NHS Scotland (n.d.). Advanced practice toolkit Available from: Advanced practice toolkit | Turas | Learn. (Accessed 24/11/2025).

NMC (2025a). Advanced Practice review. Available from www.nmc.org.uk/standards/future-standards/advanced-practice-review/?utm_source=Nursing%20and%20Midwifery%20Council&utm_medium=email&utm_campaign=14930658_20250318%20-%20Advanced%20Practice%20Principles%20%28Community%20of%20interest%29&dm_i=129A,8W0KI,UWNSIT,111D32,1 (Accessed 24/11/2025).

NMC (2025b). *Principles for advanced practice.* London: NMC.

NMC (2025c). Stakeholder engagement. Available from: www.nmc.org.uk/standards/future-standards/advanced-practice-review/stakeholder-engagement/ (Accessed 24/11/2025).

Nursing and Midwifery Council. (2002). *Annual Report and Accounts 2001–2002.*

Nursing and Midwifery Council (2010). The Proposed Framework for the Standards for Post Registration Nursing. NMC.

Nursing Midwifery Council (2018) The Code: Professional Standards of Practice and Behaviour for Nurses, Midwives and Nursing Associates. NMC.

Palmer, W., Julian S., & Vaughan L. (2023). *Independent Report on the Regulation of Advanced Practice in Nursing and Midwifery.* London: The Nuffield Trust.

Rafferty, A. (1996). *The Politics of Nursing Knowledge.* London: Routledge.

Royal College of Emergency Medicine (n.d.). RCEM Emergency Medicine ACP Credentialling. Available from: RCEM Emergency Medicine ACP Credentialing – RCEM (Accessed 24/11/2025).

Scottish Government (2017). Transforming nursing, midwifery and health professions roles: advanced nursing practice. Available from: Transforming nursing, midwifery and health professions roles: advance nursing practice – gov.scot (Accessed 24/11/2025).

Scottish Government (2021). Advanced nursing practice – transforming nursing roles: Phase two. Available from Advanced nursing practice - transforming nursing roles: phase two - gov.scot (Accessed 24/11/2025).

Scottish Government (2025). Transforming Roles paper 9: allied health professions advanced practice. Available from: Transforming Roles paper 9: allied health professions advanced practice - gov.scot (Accessed 24/11/2025).

Skills England (n.d.). Advanced Clinical Practitioner (integrated degree). Available from: Advanced clinical practitioner (integrated degree) / Skills England. (Accessed 25/11/25).

Stocks, M. (2024). A Hundred Years of District Nursing. London: Routledge.

Webster, C. (2002). *The National Health Service: A Political History.* Oxford: Oxford University Press.

PART 1

Clinical skills

CHAPTER 2

Consultation skills

Victoria M. Lack

The ability to carry out a competent consultation involves more than the capacity to take an accurate history, perform a physical assessment, make a differential diagnosis and devise a plan of action. It requires the ability to gain an understanding of what the patient needs and wants from the encounter, an awareness of hidden agendas and the competence to conclude the consultation when both patient and clinician are in agreement about a plan of action. It is also about being able to identify 'red flags', being safe and using current evidence-based practice. It is where the clinician can incorporate something of themselves into the discussion, in the way they listen, respond, perform any physical examination and plan care with the patient. This is the 'art' of consulting, and every clinician will have their own style. In this chapter the nature of the consultation is investigated, to explore the art as well as the science. Relevant consultation theory and models are discussed, as well as practical ways of enabling a successful consultation in order to ensure the best possible outcomes for patient and clinician. In addition, remote methods of consulting are discussed, as these have become increasingly prevalent in the last 15 years.

Learning outcomes

At the conclusion of this chapter you will be able to:

- Discuss consultation theory with reference to a selection of recognised models.
- Consider ways in which to develop your consultation skills.
- Reflect on changes in methods of consultation and how this is affecting your practice now and in the future.

Background

The definition of the consultation can be described as 'the act of discussing something with someone or a group of people, before making a decision about it' (Oxford Learner's

DOI: 10.4324/9781003609049-4

Dictionary, no date). It is not therefore limited to clinical environments, but can be about anything where a decision needs to be made. In the clinical setting, doctors are traditionally seen as the clinicians who undertake consultations, but the ability to assess a patient's problems and needs is an essential skill in all health professions (McGee, 2009). Maguire and Pitceathly (2002) indicate that doctors with good consultation skills are able to identify patients' problems more accurately; patients are better satisfied with the process and have a greater understanding of their condition. Patients are therefore more likely to follow the recommended treatment. It also appears that good consultation skills increase job satisfaction for the practitioner (Maguire and Pitceathly, 2002). It could be extrapolated from this that any health professional with good consultation skills will perform better.

Outside of medical practice by doctors, the term 'consultation' is not often used. The Multiprofessional Framework for Advanced Practice (Centre for Advancing Practice, 2025), does not specifically refer to 'consultation skills' when describing the competencies required by Advance Practitioners (APs) . However, within the clinical practice pillar, Competency 1.4 states that APs should be able to:

> work in partnership with individuals, families, and carers, using a range of assessment methods as appropriate (for example history-taking; holistic assessment; identifying risk factors; mental health assessments; requesting, undertaking, and/or interpreting diagnostic tests; and conducting health needs assessments)
>
> (NHS England, 2025:p.13)

In competency 1.5, the Multiprofessional Framework states that APs should be able to demonstrate effective communication skills, supporting people in making decisions and planning care. Therefore the discussion and decision-making aspects of the consultation are covered. What is perhaps missing is the 'art' of the consultation itself. The Core Capabilities for Advanced Clinical Practitioners (Nurses) working in General Practice/Primary Care in England (Health Education England et al., 2020) does include the word 'consult' in Capability 1: Communication and Consultation skills. In point 'g' it says the Advanced Clinical Practitioner (ACP) must:

> Consult in a highly organised and structured way, with professional curiosity as required, whilst understanding the constraints of the time limited nature of general practice/primary care consultations and ensure communication is safe and effective.
>
> (Health Education England, RCGP and Skills for Health, 2020:p.18)

This brings the concept of professional curiosity into the frame: which is part of the 'art' of the consultation. However, it then seems to back away from allowing this freedom, by adding 'as required' and stating that time is limited. In Capability 2 (practicing holistically to personalise care and promote public and person health) point 'h' states that ACPs must engage people in shared decision making about their care, through various techniques including supporting people to express their ideas, concerns and expectations, motivational interviewing and other methods. Perhaps because General Practitioners (GPs) are traditionally the clinicians that carry out what we understand to be consultations, the Royal College of General Practitioners (RCGPs) see the ability to consult as being an essential skill for ACPs working in primary care and call it as such. It is interesting that time is brought up by the RCGP, in acknowledgement that GP consultations are traditionally very short. In the Nursing and Midwifery Council (NMC) document 'Principles for Advanced Practice' (NMC 2025), the NMC states that advanced-level practitioners should be able to make complex and evidence-based decisions. It does not specifically mention the ability to gather information or to plan care (NMC, 2025). Neither is there any mention of the ability to carry out a consultation. However, the document is concerned only with principles and there may be more specific guidance around consultation skills at a later date.

It does appear there is a reticence in using the word 'consultation' in relation to non-doctors' clinical practice, in favour of discussing elements within that consultation such as communication skills, clinical decision making and care planning. Pendleton, a GP, in his book *The New Consultation*, calls the consultation the central act of medicine which deserves to be understood (Pendleton et al., 2003). If the assumption is made that what ACPs are doing a large part of the time is practising medicine, in the broadest sense of the word, then it is nonetheless important that ACPs learn about the 'art and science' of the consultation and how to put it into practice.

Activity 1

If you were creating a competency framework for Advanced Clinical Practitioners, how would you write a competency around the ability to perform a consultation?

Models of Consultation

Because doctors, and especially GPs, are traditionally involved in undertaking consultations, research into the consultation, and the development of consultation models, has been undertaken by doctors. This may change with the increasing numbers of non-doctors seeing people with undifferentiated diagnoses. However, much of what is discussed in the training of GP registrars is transferable to the advanced practitioner in primary or secondary care. Several well-recognised models used by doctors and other clinicians will now be discussed.

The traditional medical model focuses on tasks to be done:

> The patient says what their symptoms are;
> The clinician asks questions and examines the patient;
> The clinician says what the problem is and pronounces a treatment;
> The patient goes away.
>
> (Moulton, 2007:p.14)

This approach works very well in situations where there is a clear problem and a clear answer. To take a real-life example: a young person presents with a pain in between the ribs, which is worse on coughing. The patient has had an acute cough and has strained the intercostal muscles, resulting in muscular pain. The clinician gives a reason for the pain and advises about pain relief. The patient is happy with the explanation and advice given and goes away.

However if, as happened in reality, the patient then asked 'could this have anything to do with anxiety'? and then says they are getting short of breath with it as well (which had not been mentioned earlier), the medical model then breaks down as the patient has not accepted the treatment and gone away; they are asking for more. At this point the clinician has a decision to make; they can either dismiss the question, or try and find out the reason for it. This may open up a whole new agenda. This is probably the correct thing to do – and is mentioned in the RCGP capabilities around having curiosity. However, the capabilities say that time is also important, and the clinician needs to be mindful that by asking the question the consultation will take longer. The advantage of the medical model then is that it is usually quick and therefore many patients can be seen in 10-minute slots. It works if the perspective of the doctor and patient are the same but does not work, as in the example above, if there is a difference in the perception and understanding of the symptom(s) between the patient and doctor.

GP academics and researchers have recognised for many years that the medical model will not work for more complex issues and have advocated for a more 'patient-centred model'. McWhinney in 1998 discussed an approach called 'patient centred interviewing' to distinguish it from the doctor-led approach of the medical model. Their disease-illness model provides a way of putting this concept into practice, as in Figure 2.1.

In this, the doctor (or other clinician) comes with their agenda: i.e. to put together the symptoms and signs from their history and examination, in order to find out the particular disease process. The patient comes with their agenda, which is the experience of illness: how they are feeling physically and emotionally; what their concerns are about this, and what they hope to get from the consultation. The clinician's job is to put this together and explain the diagnosis and a plan of care that the patient

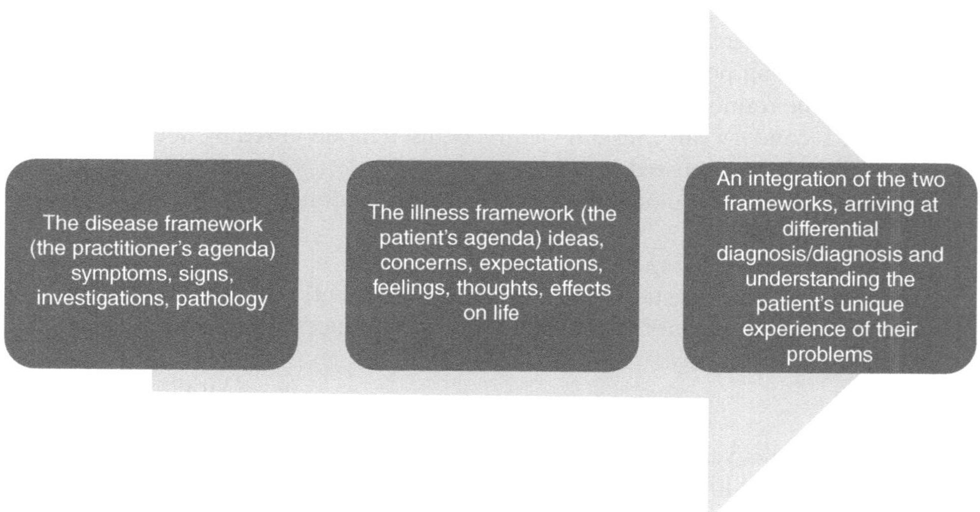

Figure 2.1 The disease illness model, adapted from McWhinney (1998)

can understand and agree with. In *The New Consultation* published initially in 2003, Pendleton, a GP, builds on the patient-centred model. He said that GPs needed to (Pendleton et al., 2003):

(1) Understand the problem
(2) Understand the patient
(3) Share understanding
(4) Share decisions and responsibility
(5) Maintain the relationship
(6) ... and do all this within the allocated time!

The above list emphasises the need for a shared understanding between patient and clinician. Broken down a little further, there are tasks to be accomplished at each stage of the list. In order to understand the patient's problem, the clinician needs to understand its nature and history, its aetiology and its effects on the patient. The clinician also needs to understand the patient: their experience of the illness or problem and also the effects it is having on the patient and their life. It is also important to explore what ideas they have about their illness, and what expectations they have from the consultation. The second task is to achieve a shared understanding about the problem and about options for management according to the best evidence available. Task three is then to help the patient choose the most appropriate course of action according to the options open to them. Task four is to agree on the appropriate responsibilities and agree on targets, monitoring and follow up. Finally, the clinician needs to consider potential problems that the patient may face and risk factors that may impede a positive outcome to the consultation. The clinician should try to encourage the patient towards as good health as is possible through health promotion advice. This model focuses on understanding the patient and their problem, in order to enable what we may now call 'person-centred care'.

Roger Neighbour, another GP, in his well-known book *The Inner Consultation* (Neighbour, 2005) discusses five checkpoints in the process of the consultation:

(1) Connecting with the patient – The clinician acts, listens and asks questions in such a way that the patient feels able to talk and discuss the issue.
(2) Summarising – This is where the clinician summarises what the patient has said and checks that they have understood.
(3) Handover – This is where the clinician discusses with the patient what is to be the plan of action and both agree on what will happen next.
(4) Safety netting – The clinician ensures that there is nothing that has been left out from the consultation; no other symptoms or factors which need to be considered. The clinician also ensures safety by discussing with the patient what to do if things do not go as expected and there is a worsening of the symptoms and/or condition.
(5) Housekeeping – This checkpoint is very important for the clinician. This is essentially about time for the clinician to consider whether they have done everything as well as can be done; that all bases have been covered. It is also time to recover from a bad consultation and ensure that the clinician is fit to go on and deal with another patient.

Neighbour also discusses the concept that most GPs will have 'two heads' during the consultation and that there will be an inner and an outer consultation taking place; hence the name of his book. The organiser 'head' is the intellectual part of the brain which takes on the 'managerial' role in the consultation. The second head, the 'responder', keeps track of emotions, sensations and feelings during the consultation and will respond to more emotional cues from the patient. Neighbour indicates it is desirable to have both 'heads' on during the consultation so both practical and emotional needs of the patient will be addressed.

The Calgary Cambridge model Kurtz & Silverman (1996) is commonly used in medical and ACP training. It is again a five-step process, as represented diagrammatically in Figure 2.2:

Unlike other models, the Calgary Cambridge model begins before initial contact with the patient is made. In 'Initiating the Session' the clinician prepares for the consultation, which should involve looking at the patient's notes (if available) to gain insight into the patient's medical history, current medication, social circumstances, any safeguarding issues and reason for the last consultation. Questions to answer would be:

Has the patient consulted about this problem before – was it in person or remotely?
What was the outcome, what treatments were prescribed/recommended?
Is the patient a regular attender, or have they not been seen for years?

The above questions are of vital importance; if treatments have already been tried (and failed) then the problem needs serious re-consideration, especially if it was previously dealt with remotely. In addition, the patient who rarely attends should raise concern: it is likely to be something significant that brings them here today. Other preparation includes ensuring there are enough chairs (if a carer/relative/friend is going to be

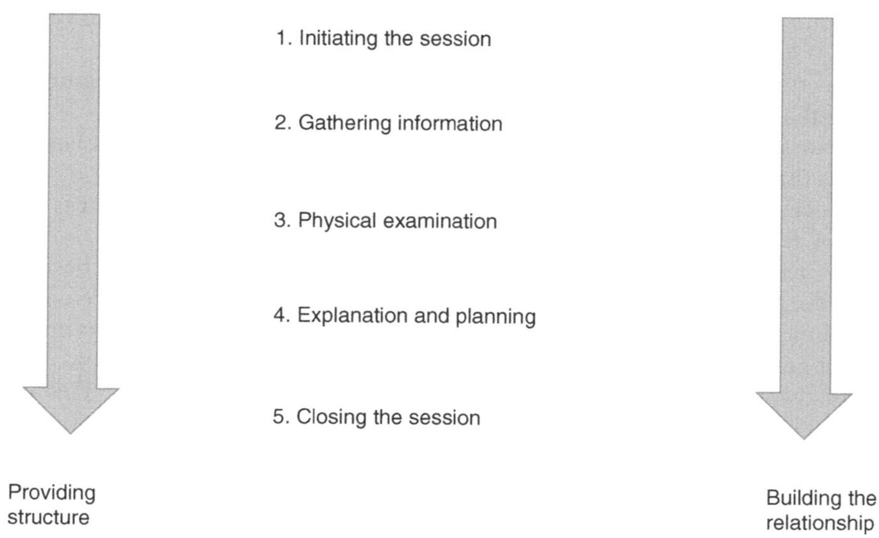

Figure 2.2 The Calgary Cambridge Model adapted from Kurtz & Silverman (1996)

present), that the right equipment is available, that translation services are available or a chaperone is available if this is indicated from the notes or appointment list.

The Gathering Information step is similar to the Pendleton model in that the patient's perspective is highlighted. After any physical examination, the fourth step, Explanation and Planning, like the other models discussed, talks about achieving a shared understanding and decision-making process. The fifth part, Closing the Session, should then be the tying up of any loose ends and ensuring that there is mutual understanding. The other distinctive part of this model are the two downward arrows: Providing structure to the consultation is the job of the clinician: The patient may be roaming in the history and bringing in a lot of information which may not be connected together. It is the role of the clinician to make sense of this information, to order it and keep the discussion on track and pay attention to the time. The right- hand arrow, building the relationship, is where the clinician's communication and therapeutic skills come into play, to ensure the patient feels listened to and understood, and enabling the patient to be involved in the process.

The above three models have many similarities and some unique points which can be used to enable a 'good' consultation. A final model, from Stewart et al. (1995), brings most of these elements together and also encourages the clinician to look at the context in which the patient exists, which may be lacking from other models. This patient-centred model is outlined diagrammatically in Figure 2.3:

This model incorporates most of the elements of the other models, but encourages the clinician to consider the social and environmental context in which the patient exists.

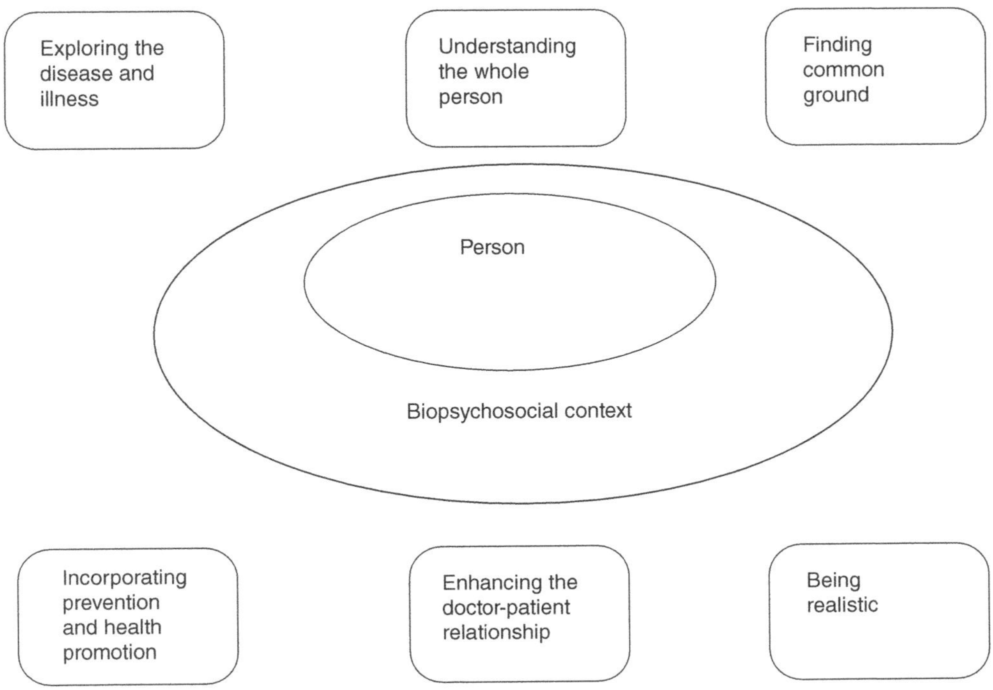

Figure 2.3 The patient-centred model from Stewart et al. (2003)

A patient presenting with pneumonia who lives with a partner who can monitor the patient, enable them to take their medication, provide supportive care and pick up the phone if the patient deteriorates is a very different prospect from the patient who lives alone in temporary accommodation, who does not have anyone to help care for them or to take action if the clinical situation worsens. As with Pendleton and the concerns around time constraints, there is a reminder to be realistic: Many thangs patients may raise may not be clinical and will not be in the clinician's remit to solve: An individual who is anxious and stressed with a low mood because they have lost their job is an issue that medicine alone cannot resolve. We can empathise and listen, but fundamentally we can rarely change people's lives.

The above models have much to inform the advanced practitioner. McWhinney's disease-illness model is a reminder that patients come with their own agenda. Pendleton's summary of tasks helps us to explore the patient's perception. The housekeeping task of Neighbour's model is essential in maintaining efficacy and preserving the well-being of the practitioner. The Calgary Cambridge model stresses the importance of preparation, which will alert the practitioner if a patient has consulted before about the same problem, but has not been helped. Finally the patient-centred model reminds the clinician to see the patient in the context of their environment.

Practical application of consultation theory

Developing consultation skills allows the clinician to implement a range of styles to suit individual patients and circumstances. This can be beneficial to the clinician and patient (Pendleton et al., 2003). The way a consultation is carried out affects the patient's adherence to treatment plans. Patients prefer, and do better, when they are involved in the medical decision-making process. There is evidence that long-term outcomes are affected by doctors using a more patient-centred approach to the consultation. It also appears that patients are less likely to sue when they feel they have been understood and respected, whatever the outcome of care (Pendleton et al., 2003). An effective consultation style is also important for job satisfaction amongst clinicians. Understanding how to make consultations a more comfortable process for clinicians and patients can decrease stress (Maguire and Pitceathly, 2002). It is also more interesting to be curious about the process: different patients may consult for similar problems many times in a week, but being able to see and understand and work with the nuances that patients bring to the problem makes the work more interesting and satisfying. As ACPs develop as clinicians, they can take from different models what enhances their practice and is helpful to them. Below are some practical applications of consultation theory which you may want to try.

It is important to let the patient tell their story. How you begin a consultation is very important. What do you normally say? Maybe it is a generic opening comment such as:

> Hello Mrs B, how are you today? or
> How can I help this morning? or
> What brings you here today?

These may seem quite neutral openers and an invitation for the patient to tell their story, but the patient may actually answer the question which may not be what you want.

For example: in answer to the last question, the answer might be: 'Well, I've come for antibiotics', which is a difficult way to start off. Moulton (2007) in her book *The Naked Consultation*, which is a practical guide to primary care consultation skills, suggests saying almost nothing, except for a polite:

> Hello, have a seat.

The patient is then obliged to make a start with no directing from the clinician. The patient may then say what they've actually been rehearsing to say in the waiting room. Try it! Of course some people will not say anything. In this case, an opening question is necessary. But even then the silence may be important. Neighbour (2005) says that the first part of the consultation is the only part that the patient has much control over: they tend to make an opening statement, which he calls the 'curtain raiser', e.g., 'I only just made it here in time'. Then the patient may say what they want: 'I just want a repeat prescription of my inhaler'. By asking an initial question, Neighbour says you may cut off the curtain raiser which may be important in finding out the mood of the patient and how the patient will behave during the consultation.

Once the patient has said their opening 'gambit' such as: 'I've got this terrible cough', they will usually go on to expand on this (Pendleton et al., 2003). They will usually talk for up to 90 seconds, at the end of which you may know most of the things which are important to the history and have a good understanding of the patient's perspective. Moulton calls these the 'golden minutes' and suggests this may continue for two to three minutes, rather than 90 seconds. She says it is very tempting to interrupt the patient during this time, to want to clarify a certain point. Try to resist the temptation to do this, but instead make encouraging noises or say throw away lines such as 'I see' or 'go on'. You may be surprised at the end how much you know and how little clarification is needed. If, however, the patient is stopped during the 'golden minutes' the patient may forget what they were saying and miss an important piece of information, they may go back to the beginning of their story or they may embellish the story to really make sure you are listening. Either way, time is not saved.

At some point however, the clinician needs to 'attend to the flow' as described in the Calgary Cambridge model. Some patients will talk for a long time and go onto subjects which are not relevant to this consultation. At this point Neighbour suggests a way to move on, without appearing that the clinician is impatient, not listening or does not care. He suggests the giving of a 'token' as he calls it. Saying something like:

> Thank you very much for telling me all this (and showing me the notes on your phone/list of concerns etc. if they have). Now I would like to ask you some questions to explore this further.

The clinician can then fill in any gaps, clarify aspects of the history, perhaps using more closed questions. Neighbour suggests almost overdoing the gratitude and the 'token' so that patients really do feel valued and that they have been listened to. This will hopefully make them forget that you have in fact interrupted them. Try this one too; it does work.

The patient's' perspective is vital in the consultation, as highlighted in the models: the patient may already have shared this with you (as long as they have been allowed to speak), but they may not. This is where following questions will come into the history taking; often known as the 'ICE' questions for Ideas, Concerns and Expectations. They may be expressed in the following ways:

What do you think may be causing this problem?
What are you concerned about today?
What are you hoping for from coming here today?

Clearly these questions need to be asked with a degree of clinical skill and judgement: it can be easy to get a glib or sarcastic answer, such as – in answer to the above questions in order:

> I don't know – you are the doctor!
> My leg is hanging off!
> To make me better of course!

However, getting an answer to these questions is really important: for example, the patient may have had similar abdominal symptoms before, which have recurred and last time it was gallstones, so they are thinking it will be this. Of course it is necessary to be aware of being led by this – it may not be gallstones this time, but it is a good starting point. They may be worried that a change in bowel habit is cancer, a concern which clearly needs to be addressed, and once the concern is 'out in the open' it is more easily discussed. Finally patients may want to know if their 'chest infection' needs specific treatment or not: often clinicians assume all patients want antibiotics; this is not the case.

It is usually time saving to ask these questions early in the consultation (if the patient has not answered them in telling their story). If a patient can tell you 'what the answer is' or give a pointer in the right direction this is very helpful. To know the patient's concerns can prevent the patient asking at the end of the consultation something like 'do you think it is cancer then doctor?', which will then need to be discussed. To know what the patient is hoping to get from the consultation is necessary to allow for the shared understanding and care planning. For example, a patient may be hoping for a 'sick note' for their back pain: they may not tell you this until the end, at which point the discussion will inevitably become longer.

When it comes to making a shared decision it is useful to be able to know whether a patient would like something to happen without having to commit to it: Neighbour gives a way to do this (Neighbour, no date). For example if a patient is complaining of chest pain, which is not obviously cardiac in origin, the clinician can look skywards and ask a rhetorical question: such as 'I'm wondering if we need to get and ECG and blood tests done'. The patient can then respond: 'Yes I would really like that' or perhaps answer no; 'I'm sure I've strained a muscle in the gym'. In this way the clinician has 'put it out there', without committing to actually doing it, which would be time consuming and unproductive if neither the patient nor the clinician feel it is necessary.

Pendleton et al. (2003) suggest asking the following questions in order to ascertain that shared understanding and decision making has been achieved:

- Do I know significantly more about the patient than before the consultation?
- Was I curious?
- Did I listen?
- Did I explore the patient's ideas, concerns, expectations, and the effects of the problem?
- Did I acknowledge the patient's viewpoint?
- Did I make an acceptable working diagnosis?

(Pendleton et al., 2003: pp.54–55)

These questions are very useful to ask in relation to self-learning or facilitating the learning of students. They can form the basis of a reflective case study, perhaps for revalidation or appraisal. The answer to the questions should, of course, be 'yes', most of the time. Yet it is probably not realistic to maintain professional curiosity over a session, days, months and years, all of the time. However, depending on the frequency and the amount of 'no's' in answer to the above questions, it may be time to get a hot drink, have lunch, have a holiday or get a new job. If the curiosity is gone, there is no caring or compassion and therefore the clinician will no longer be a safe and effective practitioner.

Activity 2

Choose two or three consultations that you have done recently and answer Pendleton's questions. Do you think that shared decision making and understanding were achieved? If not, what was the reason, and how could this be changed in the future?

Another vital aspect of the consultation, albeit a perhaps very obvious one, is that the clinician needs to have adequate knowledge and skills. It is all very well being nice and caring, but if the clinician cannot make all attempts to find out what the actual problem is, using their diagnostic skills as well as communication skills, the patient will not benefit. More about this will be discussed in the chapter on clinical decision making, but it is also worth mentioning here as it is so important. This is the 'science' of the consultation.

It is also important for clinicians to recognise what they do and do not know: Moulton (2007) discusses this as a move through four stages:

- Unconscious incompetence
- Conscious incompetence
- Conscious competence
- Unconscious competence

This is very important in relation to ACPs. A nurse or physiotherapist or paramedic may be moving from being an expert in their own field, to being a novice in advanced practice. It is therefore vital that ACPs 'know what they don't know'. This is a difficult one, because how do we recognise what we don't know? It is probably through learning more that we realise there is so much more to learn. It is also about knowing the 'red flags' and following guidelines. An example of this would be the first patient I saw with Covid-19. I did not know or suspect they had Covid (at the time this was something we thought was only happening in Wuhan and perhaps Italy). However I recognised the patient was unwell, was deteriorating and had vital signs indicating he was 'high risk of sepsis'. He was referred and treated appropriately. Another part of this is that ACPs, and all clinicians, need to be very aware of the many things they do not know and to have appropriate 'doubt'. It is fine to have conscious incompetence: patients can be discussed or referred and the ACP remains within their scope of practice. It is unconscious incompetence which is the dangerous one.

In primary care, and to a lesser extent in secondary and tertiary care, there is always an element of risk taking. In General Practice, and in a patient's home, the clinician normally lets the patient go home, or leaves the patient at home, having made a calculated decision that the patient will not deteriorate and will not require urgent medical attention. It is not common in General Practice or in a person's home to have sophisticated testing equipment available, so much is left to the traditional history-taking and examination skills of the clinician. Of course, there is also risk with discharging patients from Accident and Emergency Departments, Outpatient Departments or a ward. Pendleton et al. (2003) write about sharing decisions and responsibility whereas Neighbour (2005) writes about safety netting. These are two slightly different approaches to the end of a consultation.

Moulton (2007) indicated her first GP trainer told her that out of 20 patients in a morning surgery, 19 will probably have a trivial problem where it doesn't really matter what you do or don't do, so long as you don't cause them active harm. The 20th patient will have something wrong with them. The problem is working out which patient that is. Sometimes it will have been impossible to have predicted which patient with minor symptoms turns out to have a major problem, so it is essential to have a 'safety net' for both patient and clinician to ensure as far as possible that patients do not fall too far.

Moulton identifies three parts to safety netting:

1. Tell the patient what you think is wrong and what you expect to happen
2. Tell the patient how they would know if you are wrong
3. Tell the patient what they should do then.

(Moulton, 2007)

Neighbour (2005) suggests that a good test of whether your safety net is adequate is when you come to write it down. This should be in the Plan. If you are unable to document answers to the three questions above according to what you told the patient, then you probably did not explain clearly enough. The responsibility for decisions, as highlighted by Pendleton, needs to be shared; we cannot, nor should we, do everything for the patient. If a patient has mental capacity and chooses not to take the advice or treatment on offer, then that is their decision. Our job is to ensure that the patient has understood the rationale for the plan and the consequences of not doing it.

Activity 3

Choose several consultation notes to review against Moulton's (2007) checklist for 'safety netting'. To what extent did you provide the information she suggests should be given? How can you ensure that this information is given and understood?

Remote consultations:
Remote consultations include telephone consultations, video calls and electronic consultations. Telephone consultations have long been a part of healthcare practice, but during the Covid pandemic, the number increased dramatically. In April 2020 almost half of all appointments in General Practice took place remotely, along with a third of outpatient appointments (Morris, 2020). Since then, numbers have decreased but are still far above the pre-Covid levels. Remote consultations come with increased risk; a vital part of the consultation process is missing; the patient can be seen only via a camera or not at all. Physical examination is not possible. Consultation skills are of even more importance. Roger Neighbour talks about having 'digital warmth' in remote consultations (Neighbour, 2020). It is more difficult for the patient to know that the clinician is listening and that they care, so it is necessary to make extra effort to demonstrate this. This can be done by good preparation – as in the Calgary Cambridge model, looking at the notes prior to consultation and then discussing this with the patient, which will show that the clinician has already made an effort to help. Neighbour also reminds us to have a 'clear mindset', that the clinician should not try to do anything else while listening to the patient, although this may be tempting as the patient in a phone consultation cannot actually see if you are paying attention or not. Finally he talks about giving the patient metaphorical 'receipts' such as 'can you tell me more about the rash you mentioned' (Neighbour, 2020). This reassures the patient that you have listened and understood and want to know more.

Newer and less familiar still are asynchronous consultations; those done remotely via online platforms. In these cases there is no direct contact between the clinician and patient at all. From October 2025 every GP practice in England has been required to have an online consultation platform for the duration of their office hours for non-urgent request issues (NHS England, 2025). Whether this method of communication actually fits the definition of a consultation, and many online consultations may only be requests for repeat prescriptions or more administrative tasks, there are medical issues that are managed without direct contact between patient and clinician. In these cases all the skills and style of the clinician in listening and asking questions are taken away as well as the physical assessment element. The patient also needs to be eloquent enough to get their point across through the written word.

Finally, Artificial Intelligence (AI) may come to help all clinicians in their consultations. There are AI systems that will write the consultation notes for the clinician: it can be built to work for different clinicians requiring different types of notes; e.g., summaries or full transcripts. The companies providing these platforms argue that by having AI write the notes, the clinician can pay full attention to the patient, thereby improving the consultation. Time will tell if this is the case, and whether patients and clinicians will find it beneficial.

Activity 4
How do you think using AI to document your consultation may affect the way you carry out the consultation?

Conclusion

The consultation has been a neglected area of advanced practice; it appears that important competency documents for ACPs do not recognise that the consultation itself is an essential part of advanced clinical practice. However, it is argued in this chapter that this assumption is wrong. As advanced practice involves seeing more complex patients, where the diagnosis may be unknown or uncertain, it is essential that ACPs have the necessary consultation skills to meet this challenge. Lack of formal recognition of the skills required could lead to unsafe practice. Fortunately there is much written on consultation skills for GPs. ACPs can make much use of the experience and knowledge obtained by GPs in this area and adapt this information for use in their own practice. In the future it is desirable that ACPs create and add to the body of knowledge around consultation skills.

References

Health Education England, RCGP and Skills for Health (2020) *Core capabilities framework for Advanced Clinical Practice (Nurses) working in General Practice/Primary Care in England*. Health Education England.

Kurtz, S.M. and Silverman, J.S. (1996) The Calgary-Cambridge Observation Guides: an aid to defining the curriculum and organising the teaching in Communication Training Programmes. *Medical Education*, *30*, 83–89.

Maguire, P. and Pitceathly, C. (2002) Key communication skills and how to acquire them. *British Medical Journal*, *325*(7366), 697–700.

McGee, P. (Ed.) (2009) *Advanced Practice in Nursing and the Allied Health Professions (3rd Edition)*. Oxford: Wiley-Blackwell.

McWhinney, I. (1998) in Silverman, J., Kurtz, S. and Draper, J (2005). *Skills for Communicating with Patients*. Radcliffe Medical: Abdingdon.

Morris, J. (2020) *The remote care revolution in the NHS: Understanding impacts and attitudes*. Available at www.nuffieldtrust.org.uk/resource/the-remote-care-revolution-in-the-nhs-understanding-impacts-and-attitudes (Accessed 5th November 2025).

Moulton, L. (2007) *The Naked Consultation*. Abingdon: Radcliffe.

Neighbour, R. (n.d.) Lecture on Consultation Skills. Leeds.

Neighbour, R. (2005) *The Inner Consultation*. Abingdon: Radcliffe.

Neighbour, R. (2020) *Creating digital warmth in remote consultations, with Roger Neighbour.* Available at: www.youtube.com/watch?v=VAQE9RTgLGc (Accessed 5th November 2025).

NHS England (2025) *Millions more online consultation submissions by patients to practices in September.* Available at www.england.nhs.uk/2025/10/millions-more-online-consultation-submissions-by-patients-to-practices-in-september/ (Accessed 4th November 2025).

NMC (2025) *Principles for advanced practice*. Available at: www.nmc.org.uk/standards/guidance/advanced-practice-principles/ . (Accessed 4th November 2025).

Oxford Learners' Dictionary (no date). Available at www.oxfordlearnersdictionaries.com/definition/american_english/consultation (Accessed 5th November 2025).

Pendleton, D., Schofield, T., Tate, P. and Havelock, P. (2003) *The New Consultation: Developing Doctor – Patient Communication*. Oxford: Oxford University Press.

Stewart, M., Brown, J.B., Weston,W.W., McWhinney, I.R., McWilliam, C.L. and Freeman, T.R. (2003). *Patient-centered Medicine, Transforming the Clinical Method (2nd Edition)*. Oxford: Radcliffe Medical Press.

The Centre for Advancing Practice (2025) *Multi-professional framework for advanced practice in England*. NHS England.

CHAPTER 3

Clinical decision-making

Siobhan Hicks

Introduction

Clinical decision making is an integral part of clinical practice. One of the vital functions of an Advanced Practitioner (AP) is to be able to differentiate between patients that need more urgent treatment and assessment from those that don't. Clinical decision making is a learned skill, which is developed alongside increasing knowledge and experience. It appears different clinicians use various methods to make decisions, albeit mostly unconsciously, and the same clinician may use different methods depending on the complexity of the situation and the familiarity of the clinician with it. What does seem to be apparent is that practitioners require a substantial knowledge of the subject area before safe and effective decisions can be made. It is therefore necessary to have access to resources to facilitate decision making as not all knowledge necessary can be retained. Clinical decision making is not only about the individual clinician and their skills; it is also about the ability of the organisation as a whole to ensure clinical decisions are made with the most up-to-date evidence available so that quality and equality are attained. This concept, embedded in clinical governance, will be examined in the second half of the chapter.

Learning outcomes

At the conclusion of this chapter, you will be able to:

- Discuss the steps involved in clinical decision making
- Explore what knowledge is necessary in order to make effective clinical decisions
- Understand the importance of clinical governance in terms of client safety and professional development
- Discuss the benefits of clinical supervision within the clinical governance agenda

DOI: 10.4324/9781003609049-5

Background

In order to engage in appropriate clinical decision making, APs need to have subject-specific knowledge as a prerequisite. The seminal model by Haynes et al. (2002) cites that clinical expertise involves knowledge of the patient's clinical condition, knowledge of research-based evidence, and patient preferences. Thompson et al. (2013) agree that combining clinical expertise, patient preferences, and research evidence is paramount.

Therefore, clinical decision making involves research-based knowledge, physical assessment skills, and communication. However, clinical decision making does not just require knowledge. It requires the application of that knowledge in order to formulate a diagnosis and plan of action in areas where nurses and other healthcare professionals (HCPs) would traditionally defer to a medical colleague. According to Bloom's Taxonomy (Bloom, 1956), diagnosis is an analytical skill involving critical thinking.

Historically, this was reflected in the Nursing and Midwifery Council's (NMC) guidance on the training of Advanced Nurse Practitioners (ANPs), which emphasised the need for 'M-level thinking' (NMC, 2005). At that time, however, most nurses in England were educated at diploma level, with graduate entry into the profession only introduced in 2013. As a result, opportunities to develop critical thinking skills were limited, and such competencies were neither systematically embedded in curricula nor formally assessed prior to this transition. However, the question remains: How can nurses move from a level of thinking that involves knowledge and comprehension, onto a level where they are able to apply knowledge and begin to analyse that knowledge? For example, where they are using the skill of critical thinking? This important issue may be less so for other non-medical clinicians, as their training is usually at degree level, where they are often taught decision-making models and how to think critically.

Bloom's (1956) theoretical model analysis shows the cognitive functions involved in decision making. The functions are classified into six dynamic levels of increasing complexity as shown below in Table 3.1.

There is ordinarily a sequential progression from knowledge to comprehension, to application, to analysis, to synthesis, and finally to evaluation. Therefore, in order to be able to make a competent clinical diagnosis the clinician must be able to:

- Obtain and appreciate the meaning of symptoms and signs of the patient
- Identify the appropriate organ system/s involved in disease
- Speculatively identify the possible pathological processes that is/are occurring
- Know how to differentiate one pathological process from the other
- Know from epidemiology the most likely causes of particular pathological processes
- Evaluate all pieces of information available and decide on the likely cause and course of illness

The decision-making process

Interest in how nurses make decisions dates back to the seminal work of Patricia Benner in the late 1980s (Benner and Tanner, 1987). Benner argued that nurses tend towards a humanistic–intuitive approach, whereas others such as Bench-Capon (1990) propose a more systematic model. These approaches were largely based on work with general nurses, and APs may need to apply alternative or additional methods.

Table 3.1 Cognitive Functions Involved in Clinical Decision Making

Cognitive level	*Keywords*	*Example*
1. Knowledge	Recognition, recall	Recognition of symptoms and signs
2. Comprehension	Translation	Assigning signs and symptoms to systems, i.e. vomiting and diarrhoea to gastrointestinal
3. Application	Relate, transfer associate	Relating signs and symptoms to pathological conditions, i.e. diarrhoea to gastro-enteritis or colitis
4. Analysis	Distinguish, discriminate	Picking out the specific (which are key disease indicators) from the non-specific
5. Synthesis	Formulate, combine	Putting features together into a recognisable pattern for a specific condition or conditions
6. Evaluation	Validate, argue, reconsider, appraise	Checking if the diagnosis explains all signs and symptoms, identifying any symptoms that are not easily explained and the features of the diagnosed condition that are missing

Adapted from Bloom (1956).

In studies of how health professionals in general make clinical decisions, two main models emerge. In the hypothetico-deductive method, the clinician derives hypotheses from the patient's presenting complaint that drive data collection and decision making (Offredy, 1998). In the pattern-matching model, clinicians use key clues to identify familiar patterns and make decisions based on previous experience with those patterns (Mandin et al., 1997). Benner's (1987) concept of intuition has also been examined separately and appears linked to the pattern-matching method, although intuition occurs largely at a subconscious level (Offredy, 1998).

Both pattern-matching and intuition rely on significant experience. Novices therefore tend to make decisions differently from experienced practitioners (Benner and Tanner, 1987). Newly qualified nurse practitioners often demonstrate this contrast when compared to their more experienced colleagues (Offredy, 1998). However, experienced APs will typically revert to the hypothetico-deductive model when faced with unfamiliar situations (Offredy, 1998).

Interestingly, research suggests that the methodology of decision making matters less than mastery of the clinical domain (Offredy, 1998). A classic article in the *British Medical Journal* by Elstein and Schwarz (2002) reviewed the literature on clinical problem solving and diagnostic decision making by doctors. They concluded that diagnostic accuracy depends less on the strategy used and more on content mastery. Experienced clinicians often use pattern recognition or knowledge retrieval, turning to deductive strategies only for complex cases. The educational implication of this finding is that problem-based learning, particularly the case study approach, benefits students by teaching them to test hypotheses before encountering real patients (Elstein and Schwarz, 2002). Since most care situations will be complex for students, educators should prioritise teaching hypothesis testing early. As clinicians gain experience, they naturally develop proficiency in pattern recognition.

Activity 1
Think of a consultation where you were able to reach a diagnosis by pattern-matching and one where you had to use a deductive approach. What resources did you need in order to achieve a diagnosis in the second case?

Clinical reasoning techniques
Skills in clinical decision making can be consciously developed through critical thinking during history taking. A useful strategy is to ask 'why' and 'what if' questions, mapping diagnostic possibilities to broaden and refine hypotheses. For the trainee or newly qualified AP, it may be helpful to record answers to these questions in a mind map, which can then be refined as more information emerges.

Take the example of a young child presenting with ear pain. The question would be 'why are they presenting with ear pain?' There could be several answers here, including otitis media, otitis externa, or any viral upper respiratory tract infection. However, if they also have fever, systemic malaise, and mastoid tenderness, the question is 'why are they unwell with the ear pain?' The diagnosis could then be refined to conditions which cause systemic upset. The next question would be 'why do they have mastoid tenderness?' and then mastoiditis needs to be considered. The 'what if?' question would be; if it was mastoiditis, what would need to happen?' The answer to this would be immediate referral to secondary care. Another structured approach is to begin with potential *red flags* and work downward to more likely but less serious conditions. In practice, less experienced APs may find it safer to ask, 'What is the worst thing this could be?' and rule this diagnosis out, before moving onto more likely and less severe conditions. Of course, if the worst-case scenario cannot be safely ruled out, the clinician needs to proceed with this as the hypothesis and take immediate action to refer to a setting where the hypothesis can be safely ruled out or managed if the worst-case scenario does turn out to be correct.

This reflective approach not only strengthens diagnostic accuracy but also encourages clinicians to remain alert to subtle or atypical presentations. By consciously applying such reasoning techniques, practitioners can transition more confidently from novice to expert decision makers (Benner and Tanner, 1987; Offredy, 1998).

Patient-shared decision making
Shared decision making is a collaborative process in which treatment choices are agreed upon between clinician and patient. The aim is to select options that maximise the likelihood of positive health outcomes while minimising risks. This process also helps detect when information does not fit expected patterns, prompting clinicians to reconsider assumptions. When deciding on a plan of action, often no active treatment is needed. For example, when a young child presents with a viral upper respiratory tract infection, parents may expect antibiotics. However, a clear explanation of the illness, reassurance about its natural course, and advice on analgesia can usually enable the clinician and parents to come to a shared decision about how to manage the illness, which will include providing safety-netting advice and the option to return if symptoms worsen, to support parental confidence in the decision.

Shared decision making therefore integrates patient preferences with research evidence and clinical expertise, aligning with National Institute for Health and Care Excellence (NICE) guidance (NICE, 2021). Tools such as the STEPS framework, discussed later (Pegler and Underhill, 2005), can further support practitioners in assessing whether an intervention is safe, tolerable, effective, affordable, and simple to use.

Emotional intelligence

Emotions influence how clinicians think, behave, and pay attention in practice. Effectively managing these emotions is essential for safe, confident decision making. Emotional intelligence (EI), the ability to recognise, understand, and regulate emotions in oneself and others, plays a crucial role in supporting effective clinical performance (Goleman, 1998). Goleman outlines five key domains of EI: self-awareness, self-regulation, motivation, empathy, and social skills. Together, these competencies enhance communication, teamwork, and problem solving, particularly in complex or high-pressure clinical settings.

Clinicians with high EI are often more confident and resilient in their decision making. They remain reflective and open to learning, which not only improves patient care but also supports professional development. Developing EI is especially valuable in advanced roles, where decisions carry significant consequences and require a balance of emotional insight and clinical judgement.

By the very nature of their work, clinicians are frequently exposed to profound, moving, and sometimes distressing experiences. These encounters can catalyse personal growth and lead to deep professional satisfaction, particularly when difficult cases are managed competently. Encouraging a sense of 'success' enhances problem-solving capabilities by fostering a strong sense of self-concept and self-efficacy (Berger, 1984). In order to make effective clinical decisions, especially in challenging situations, clinicians must believe in their own capacity to do so. Like many complex processes, proficiency in decision making relies on motivation and the ability to learn from experience. Listening, reflecting, and integrating knowledge are key steps that allow a well-considered decision to emerge.

Biases and preconceptions

Biases and assumptions can negatively influence clinical decision making. For example, a frail or thin patient may be wrongly perceived as seriously unwell or unable to perform daily activities, when this may not be the case. Such subjective impressions risk leading to misdiagnosis or inappropriate care. To counteract these risks, clinicians must validate their impressions through systematic data gathering, effective interviewing, and the use of objective evidence (Thompson et al., 2013). Critical reflection and awareness of personal preconceptions are also essential in ensuring decisions are safe, balanced, and patient-centred.

Clinical governance

Clinical governance is a framework that holds healthcare organisations accountable for continuously improving service quality and safeguarding patient care. It ensures that

Table 3.2 Emotional Intelligence

Self-awareness Knowing one's internal states, preferences, resources, and intuitions	Emotional awareness: *Recognising one's emotions and their effects* Accurate self-assessment: *Knowing one's strengths and limits* Self-confidence: *A strong sense of one's self-worth and capabilities*
Self-regulation Managing one's internal impulses and resources	Self-control: *Keeping disruptive emotions and impulses in check* Trustworthiness: *Maintaining standards of honesty and integrity* Conscientiousness: *Taking the responsibility for personal performance* Adaptability: *Flexibility in handling change* Innovation: *Being comfortable with novel ideas, approaches, and new information*
Motivation Emotional tendencies that guide or facilitate reaching goals	Achievement drive: *Striving to improve or meet a standard of excellence* Commitment: *Aligning with goals of the group or organisation* Initiative: *Readiness to act on opportunities*
Personal Skills How we manage ourselves	Optimism: *Persistence in pursuing goals despite obstacles and setbacks*
Social skills	Communicating and relating to others: *Listening openly and sending convincing messages*

Source: Goleman (1998).

appropriate systems are in place to monitor practice, manage risks, and foster a culture of learning and improvement (NHS England, 2021).

For the clinician

In considering the notion of risk for the AP, it is undeniable that lifelong education, experience, and organisational support are central factors in reducing harm when making decisions in clinical practice. This means exercising professional judgement, reflecting critically on practice, and engaging in lifelong learning to maintain safe standards. Tools such as reflective records, supervision, and adherence to the NMC Code (2018) support transparency and accountability. The format for this can be flexible and may include reflective diary entries, or structured spreadsheets (see Example 1). This ongoing exercise creates a written record of knowledge and experience that can be revisited over time, supporting reflection and growth across all four pillars of advanced practice (NHS England, 2025) and the NMC revalidation process (2016). In this way, the simple act of recording consultations becomes a valuable strategy for embedding reflection, advancing professional standards, and supporting both personal and professional development as an AP.

In the words of Franklin P. Jones (unknown), 'Experience is that marvellous thing that enables you to recognize a mistake when you make it again.'

Example 1

Date	*ID*	*Age*	*Complaint*	*Diagnosis*	*Treatment*	*Referral*	*Follow up*	*Notes*
		19	Abdominal pain	? Appendicitis	Refer	Surgical team	Admitted	Appendectomy
		3	Ear pain	Viral URTI	OTC analgesia	Pharmacy	Did not reattend	
		75	Discharge from wound	Infected laparotomy wound site	Swab MC&S. Oral antibiotic	None	Did not reattend	
		8	Sore throat	Viral tonsillitis	OTC analgesia	Pharmacy	Reconsulted General Practitioner 3 days later	Given oral antibiotic. *(rationale reviewed by AP (date)*

Activity 2

How do you review your clinical decision-making skills in practice?

A wide range of evidence-based resources are available to support clinical decision making and professional development, including guidance from the *National Institute for Health and Care Excellence* (NICE, n.d.) and the *Scottish Intercollegiate Guidelines Network* (SIGN, n.d.). Modular learning opportunities are also provided by *BMJ Learning* (BMJ Learning, n.d.), while patient-focused information and professional updates can be accessed through charities such as *Diabetes UK* (Diabetes UK, n.d.) and the *National Eczema Society* (National Eczema Society, n.d.). Most recently, clinical decision support systems (CDSS) can play an important role in improving the safety and efficiency of clinical decision making by embedding evidence-based guidelines into clinical software systems. They support standardised care, enhance patient safety, and boost efficiency. However, issues like alert fatigue, workflow disruptions, and over-reliance on prompts may undermine clinical judgement and critical thinking if poorly managed (Kwon et al., 2019). This highlights the need to balance the benefits of CDSS with their risks, ensuring they support, not replace, clinical expertise.

An interesting development is the advent of pharmacists taking on more responsibility for minor ailments. This can help reduce the burden on General Practices, but it is also likely that the patients General Practitioners (GPs) and APs see will be more complex in nature. This shift requires effective collaboration between healthcare professionals, ensuring that patients receive the appropriate level of care at the right point in the system.

The overarching aim of clinical governance is to ensure that a comprehensive range of guidelines is in place to facilitate evidence-based practice. To a large extent, this aim can be achieved, leaving little justification for claiming that knowledge is unavailable to support effective clinical decision making.

For Educators

Support for educators is available through the *Association of Advanced Practice Educators* (AAPE), who work closely with the Royal College of Nursing (RCN), the RCN Nurse Practitioner Forum, and the NMC. Together, they represent a collaborative network of Higher Education Institutions (HEIs) across the United Kingdom that support educators providing advanced clinical programmes of education for nurses. Additionally, Advanced Clinical Practitioner (ACP) programme accreditation is the process by which Health Education England (HEE) (now incorporated into NHS England) evaluates and approves HEIs offering ACP master's-level programmes to ensure they meet national standards. This ensures consistency across ACP roles nationally and provides assurance to employers, patients, and regulators. It may also help ACPs meet requirements for any future statutory regulation.

For Employers

Employers have access to a range of tools that support new ways of working. The *Skills for Health* website provides information and guidance on developing competencies, frameworks, and learning and development needs for advanced practice roles (Skills for Health, n.d.). These frameworks are mapped against the *NHS Employers Terms and Conditions of Service Handbook* (NHS Employers, 2025), which incorporates the principles of clinical governance by emphasising training, competence assessment, ongoing supervision, and risk management. Importantly, these resources are free to access and available to both clinicians and employers.

Organisational clinical governance resources underpin the Four Pillars of Advanced Practice by supporting competence in clinical care, ensuring the delivery of safe, effective, and evidence-based interventions. In leadership and management, these resources provide frameworks that promote accountability, workforce development, and the implementation of new models of care. In education, they offer structured learning opportunities and facilitate competency development. Lastly, in research, they encourage the critical appraisal of practice and align service delivery with evidence-informed frameworks, ensuring continuous improvement and innovation in healthcare.

Accreditation

Accreditation is a hot topic in advanced practice for nurses because it may provide a structured way of assuring quality, safety, and public trust, all factors that are important in clinical governance. Historically, competencies for Advanced Practice were set out by the NMC (2005), CHRE (Council for Healthcare Regulatory Excellence) (2009), and the RCN (2010), who provided agreed standards that supported the development and regulation of advanced practice. The CHRE report to the four UK health departments (2009) noted that much of what was described as advanced practice was often career development rather than a fundamental departure from a profession's core practice. As such, existing standards of proficiency were considered sufficient to protect patient safety, and additional statutory regulation, including a separate register for APs, was deemed unnecessary.

However, advanced roles often extend beyond traditional nursing or allied health boundaries, incorporating elements of medical practice. This shift requires greater autonomy and accountability. In this context, it is important to recall the Bolam Test

(*Bolam v Friern Hospital Management Committee*, 1957), which highlights the duty of care to patients: if negligence occurs, practitioners are judged against the standard of a reasonably competent professional in that role i.e. another AP or a doctor.

Most recently, the NMC Principles for Advanced Practice (2025) have provided updated guidance to promote clarity, consistency, and safety in advanced nursing and midwifery roles across the UK. Developed in collaboration with professionals, employers, and the public, these principles aim to address ongoing variation in how advanced practice is defined and implemented (NMC, 2025).

At present, a dedicated advanced practice register is not expected until at least 2027/28, when there are plans to develop standards of proficiency and associated programme standards, followed by public consultation (NMC, 2024). There is accreditation for the ACP role – but it is awarded to educational programmes rather than individuals; the title itself remains unregulated. In the interim, the NMC is reviewing the *Code* and preparing transitional arrangements for advanced nurse practitioners (NMC, 2024). Reflecting this regulatory shift, the RCN halted new applications for credentialling in June 2025, with existing credentials to remain valid until November 2028 (RCN, 2025). By contrast, advanced practice roles regulated by the Health and Care Professions Council (HCPC) remain overseen within their existing statutory registration frameworks, with no additional register proposed (HCPC, 2024).

Clinical supervision

Clinical supervision is a structured process that supports safe, effective, and reflective practice within advanced roles and fits into the clinical governance agenda. When delivered well, it provides APs with opportunities for professional growth, peer support, and innovation, while also strengthening clinical governance (Skills for Health, n.d.; NHS Employers, 2025).

Supervision can take different forms, including one-to-one, group, or peer-led models. Regardless of format, it fosters critical reflection, empathy, and teamwork, which enhances both patient safety and professional development. It also aligns with the four pillars of advanced practice by supporting evidence-based clinical decisions, developing leadership skills, encouraging reflective education, and promoting enquiry into practice (NHS England, 2025). Moreover, supervision reinforces professional accountability, as outlined in the NMC Code (2018), by encouraging openness to feedback and continuous improvement. Where formal supervision is not available, APs can still benefit from peer-led reflective groups or virtual platforms to sustain these essential practices. APs should choose the method which is most appropriate for their learning and developmental needs, and what is available in clinical practice. It can still be a useful instrument for reflection, facilitating empathy and cohesion within a team.

Example 2 shows how facilitated clinical supervision managed friction within a General Practice team which could have hindered clinical decision making.

Example 2

This session was attended by four practice nurses, one ANP, four GPs and an external facilitator. A GP initiated the discussion by saying she felt under pressure and irritated by frequent interruptions to her consultations from the nurses. She felt that because of this the care she was providing in her consultations was compromised.

The main response to this was the practice nurses reminding the GP that often they were dealing with complex decisions that needed timely advice – for example, issues surrounding titration of insulin; exacerbations of Chronic Obstructive Pulmonary Disease *(COPD)/Asthma; prescribing or social issues. The other GPs and the ANP did not support the GP. In fact they were glad to be interrupted if it prevented an error being made by another practitioner or having to make another appointment for the same patient with them.*

This scenario threw light on some uncomfortable issues. It was acknowledged by the participants that the doctors were also asking for advice; not just from each other but from the nursing team, especially in areas such as chronic disease management. The workload for the on-call GP was unbalanced; causing stress to the GP and compromised care to patients.

Following discussion, it was agreed that asking for and providing help is one of the most important things a practitioner must do. The GP recognised the value of the clinical input from the nurses and that their questions were just as valid as the doctors'. The nurses appreciated the pressures that the GP was under and were able, in the end, to view this situation sympathetically. Everyone was forced to review their rationale for disturbing consultations, raising awareness of boundaries and timely interruption. The clinical supervision session was a confidential meeting; most of the partnership was present. Subsequently the on-call arrangements were reviewed and revised as a result of this session. The process demonstrated the role of supervision in highlighting professional challenges, improving team cohesion, and ultimately enhancing patient safety.

Clinical supervision acts not only as a tool for individual professional growth but also as a system-level safeguard, ensuring that high-quality, patient-centred care remains at the heart of advanced clinical practice.

Activity 3

Do you or would you engage in clinical supervision if your employer or organisation did not value its effectiveness? If not valued by your organisation, think of ways in which you could still engage in the process with your peers.

Evidence-based decisions

Evidence-based medicine (EBM) has become central to improving the quality of clinical decision making, offering a structured approach that integrates the best available research evidence with clinical expertise and patient values. Sackett et al. (1996) famously defined EBM as 'the conscientious, explicit, and judicious use of current best evidence in making decisions about the care of individual patients,' marking a shift away from reliance on tradition and unsystematic clinical experience towards a more transparent and rigorous approach.

Despite its widespread adoption, challenges remain in the practical application of EBM. Time pressures, variable access to high-quality research, and the complexity of individual patient circumstances often limit its consistent use in clinical settings (Greenhalgh et al., 2014). Moreover, concerns have been raised that an overemphasis on guideline adherence may undervalue professional judgement and the nuances of patient-centred care (Bensing, 2000).

Within the UK, EBM principles underpin national frameworks for advanced practice, with emphasis placed on critical thinking, reflective practice, and the integration of research into everyday clinical decision making (NHS England, 2021 and 2025). This ensures that APs not only deliver safe and effective care but also contribute to the ongoing development of evidence-informed healthcare.

Experience can sometimes provide a false sense of certainty and is of limited use when clinicians are faced with situations they have not previously encountered. From an evidence-based perspective, a 'good' clinical decision is one that successfully integrates four interdependent elements:

(1) **Professional expertise ('know-how' knowledge)** – The ability to draw on clinical skills, experiential learning, and professional judgement in order to guide care. For instance, research evidence may recommend a treatment approach that is unsuitable for an individual patient. Recognising such mismatches, and advocating appropriately, requires confidence, advanced knowledge, and clinical reasoning.
(2) **Available resources** – Resources for evidence-based decision making extend beyond funding to include organisational culture, access to reliable evidence, and professional support. Clinicians must weigh cost-effectiveness, particularly within Integrated Care Systems where decisions must be justified to both patients and commissioners (NHS England, 2022). Access to guidance from sources such as NICE and the Cochrane Library is essential, but the ability to critically appraise and apply this information often depends on available skills, mentorship, and professional networks. These factors ultimately determine whether research evidence can be effectively translated into patient-centred care.
(3) **Patient's informed values and preferences** – It is essential, when considering concordance with treatment or medication regimens, to listen carefully to the patient's ideas, concerns, and expectations. Tools such as the **STEPS acronym** (see Table 3.3) (Pegler and Underhill, 2005) can help assess the suitability of an intervention, but current guidance also emphasises the importance of shared decision making to ensure care aligns with patient values (NICE, 2021). By first making sense of the evidence and options, practitioners are better placed to support patients in making informed choices.
(4) **Research knowledge ('know-what' knowledge)** – The sheer volume of information now available makes navigation challenging, yet for EBM to effectively inform decision making it is vital to develop critical appraisal skills. Key considerations include:

- Understanding the difference between randomised controlled trials, observational studies, and case reports.
- Recognising what longitudinal or cohort studies involve and how they contribute to evidence over time.

Table 3.3 The STEPS Test

Safety: Remember that only limited safety information is available from prospective clinical studies and Randomised Controlled Trials. Safety data from real-life comparison studies may be more useful as these will reflect the patient population.
Tolerability: Rates of withdrawal of interventions in clinical studies can be an indicator of whether interventions have effects that will influence compliance.
Effectiveness: Consideration should be given to whether the drug/intervention works in the real world.
Price: All costs should be considered including the extra costs of titration and regular monitoring.
Simplicity of use: Frequency of administration and ease of delivery and use can mean the difference between compliance and non-compliance.

Source: Pegler and Underhill (2005).

Table 3.4 Hierarchy of Strength of Evidence Used in Grading Recommendations in NICE Clinical Guidelines (Strongest to Weakest)

1a	Evidence from systematic reviews or meta-analyses of randomised controlled trials.
1b	Evidence from at least one randomised controlled trial.
11a	Evidence from at least one controlled study without randomisation.
11b	Evidence from at least one other type of quasi-experimental study.
11	Evidence from non-experimental descriptive studies, such as case control studies.
1V	Evidence from expert committee reports or opinions or clinical experience of respected authorities.

Source: Sackett et al. (2000:172).

- Knowing how a meta-analysis is constructed and how it strengthens or limits conclusions.
- Assessing research methods, including whether the sample size was adequate to support validity.
- Identifying potential sources of bias, such as funding, questionnaire design, or conflicts of interest.

Practical tools such as the **Critical Appraisal Skills Programme (CASP) checklists** (CASP, 2023) and **NICE evidence standards** (NICE, 2021) can support clinicians in systematically applying these principles to research and practice.

Conclusion

Clinical decision making is what distinguishes APs from other practitioners, as it requires more than routine experience or familiarity with situations. It demands critical thinking, reflection, and the integration of multiple factors rather than reliance on facts alone. Good decisions balance professional expertise, patient values, available resources, and research evidence.

Clinical governance frameworks reinforce this process by ensuring that decision making remains transparent, evidence-informed, and focused on patient safety and quality improvement. For APs, this means not only applying current knowledge but also leading by example in embedding governance principles into everyday practice. By doing so, they ensure that their decisions are accountable, patient-centred, and continuously aligned with evolving professional standards.

Acknowledgment
The editor would like to thank Elaine Cockram for her contribution to the first edition of the book, we have built on her works in this new edition.

References

Association of Advanced Practice Educators (AAPE) (n.d.) *About us*. Available at: https://aape.org.uk (Accessed: 10 September 2025).
Bench-Capon, T. (1990) *Knowledge representation*. London: Harcourt Brace Jovanich.
Benner, P. and Tanner, C.A. (1987) 'How expert nurses use intuition', *American Journal of Nursing*, 87(1), pp. 23–31.
Bensing, J. (2000) 'Bridging the gap: The separate worlds of evidence-based medicine and patient-centered medicine', *Patient Education and Counseling*, 39(1), pp. 17–25.
Berger, M. (1984) 'Clinical thinking ability and nursing students', *Journal of Nursing Education*, 23(7), pp. 306–308.
Bloom, B.S. (1956) *Taxonomy of educational objectives*. Boston: Allyn and Bacon.
BMJ Learning (n.d.) *BMJ Learning*. Available at: https://new-learning.bmj.com (Accessed: 10 September 2025).
Bolam v Friern Hospital Management Committee [1957] 1 WLR 582, [1957] 2 All ER 118 (QBD).
CASP (Critical Appraisal Skills Programme) (2023) *CASP checklists*. Oxford: CASP UK. Available at: https://casp-uk.net/casp-tools-checklists/ (Accessed: 10 September 2025).
Cochrane (2025) *Cochrane Library*. Available at: www.cochranelibrary.com (Accessed: 10 September 2025).
Council for Healthcare Regulatory Excellence (2009) *Advanced practice: Report to the four UK health departments*. Available at: www.chre.org.uk (Accessed: 14 June 2011).
Diabetes UK (n.d.) *Diabetes UK: Know diabetes. Fight diabetes*. Available at: www.diabetes.org.uk (Accessed: 10 September 2025).
Elstein, A.S. and Schwartz, A. (2002) 'Evidence base of clinical diagnosis', *British Medical Journal*, 324, pp. 729–732.
Goleman, D. (1998) *Working with emotional intelligence*. New York: Bantam.
Greenhalgh, T., Howick, J. and Maskrey, N. (2014) 'Evidence based medicine: A movement in crisis?', *BMJ*, 348, g3725.
Haynes, R.B., Devereaux, P.J. and Guyatt, G.H. (2002) 'Physicians' and patients' choices in evidence based practice: Evidence does not make decisions, people do', *BMJ*, 324, p. 1350.
Health and Care Professions Council (HCPC) (2024) *Advanced practice and regulation*. Available at: www.hcpc-uk.org (Accessed: 10 September 2025).
Jones, F.P. (n.d.) wist: wish I'd said that. Available at: https://wist.info/author/jones-franklin-p/ (Accessed 7 June 2026).
Kwon, J.H., Reske, K.A., Hink, T., Jackups, R., Burnham, C.A.D. and Dubberke, E.R. (2019) 'Impact of an electronic hard-stop clinical decision support tool to limit repeat *Clostridioides difficile* toxin enzyme immunoassay testing on test utilization', *Infection Control & Hospital Epidemiology*, 40(12), pp. 1423–1426. doi:10.1017/ice.2019.275.
Mandin, H., Jones, A. and Woloschuk, W. (1997) 'Helping students learn to think like experts when solving clinical problems', *Academic Medicine*, 72(3), pp. 173–179.
National Eczema Society (n.d.) *National Eczema Society*. Available at: https://eczema.org (Accessed: 10 September 2025).

National Institute for Health and Care Excellence (NICE) (n.d.) *Guidance*. Available at: www.nice.org.uk/guidance (Accessed: 10 September 2025).

National Institute for Health and Care Excellence (NICE) (2021) *The NICE strategy 2021 to 2026: Dynamic, collaborative, excellent*. London: NICE. Available at: https://static.nice.org.uk/NICE%20strategy%202021%20to%202026%20-%20Dynamic,%20Collaborative,%20Excellent.pdf (Accessed: 10 September 2025).

NHS Employers (2025) *NHS terms and conditions of service handbook*. Available at: www.nhsemployers.org/ (Accessed: 10 September 2025).

NHS England (2021) The Matron's Handbook: Governance, patient safety and quality. Available at: www.england.nhs.uk/mat-transformation/matrons-handbook/governance-patient-safety-and-quality/ (Accessed: 10 September 2025).

NHS England (2022) *Thriving places: Guidance on the development of place-based partnerships as part of statutory integrated care systems*. Available at: www.england.nhs.uk/wp-content/uploads/2021/06/B0660-ics-implementation-guidance-on-thriving-places.pdf (Accessed: 10 September 2025).

NHS England (2025) *Multi-professional framework for advanced practice in England*. Available at: https://advanced-practice.hee.nhs.uk/multi-professional-framework-for-advanced-practice/ (Accessed: 10 September 2025).

Nursing and Midwifery Council (2005) *Implementation of a framework for the standard for post registration nursing*. Retrieved from www.aape.org.uk/news-events/regulator-updates/ (Accessed 7 June 2026).

Nursing and Midwifery Council (2016) *Revalidation: The process to maintain nurse and midwife registration*. Available at: www.nmc.org.uk/revalidation/ (Accessed: 10 September 2025).

Nursing and Midwifery Council (2018) *The Code: Professional standards of practice and behaviour for nurses, midwives and nursing associates*. London: NMC. Available at: www.nmc.org.uk/standards/code (Accessed: 10 September 2025).

Nursing and Midwifery Council (2024) *Advanced practice review*. Available at: www.nmc.org.uk/standards/future-standards/advanced-practice-review/ (Accessed: 10 September 2025).

Nursing and Midwifery Council (2025) *Principles for advanced practice*. Available at: www.nmc.org.uk (Accessed: 10 September 2025).

Offredy, M. (1998) 'The application of decision making concepts by nurse practitioners in general practice', *Journal of Advanced Nursing*, 28(5), pp. 988–1000.

Peglar, S. and Underhill, J. (2005) 'Evaluating promotional material from industry: An evidence based approach', *The Pharmaceutical Journal*, 274, pp. 271–274.

Royal College of Nursing (2010) *Advanced nurse practitioners – An RCN guide to the advanced nurse practitioner role, competencies and programme accreditation*. London: RCN.

Royal College of Nursing (RCN) (2025) *Credentialing for advanced level nursing practice*. Available at: www.rcn.org.uk/Professional-Development/Professional-services/Credentialing (Accessed: 10 September 2025).

Sackett, D.L., Richardson, S.W., Rosenberg, W. and Haynes, R.B. (2000) *Evidence-based medicine: How to practice and teach EBM*. London: Churchill Livingstone.

Sackett, D.L., Rosenberg, W.M.C., Gray, J.A.M., Haynes, R.B. and Richardson, W.S. (1996) 'Evidence based medicine: What it is and what it isn't', *BMJ*, 312(7023), pp. 71–72.

Scottish Intercollegiate Guidelines Network (SIGN) (n.d.) *Guidelines*. Available at: www.sign.ac.uk (Accessed: 10 September 2025).

Skills for Health (n.d.) *Skills for health*. Available at: www.skillsforhealth.org.uk/ (Accessed: 10 September 2025).

Thompson, C., Aitken, L., Doran, D. and Dowding, D. (2013) 'An agenda for clinical decision making and judgement in nursing research and education', *International Journal of Nursing Studies*, 50(12), pp. 1720–1726. doi: 10.1016/j.ijnurstu.2013.05.003.

CHAPTER 4

Planning care

Ruth Walters

Introduction

The aim of this chapter is to explore the use of planning care in promoting health and well-being by empowering patients and encouraging shared decision making within the context of advanced practice. The challenge facing healthcare professionals in planning effective care with patients must not be underestimated and the process requires the utilisation of a range of skills and competencies. In considering care planning for advanced practitioners it is important to understand that aspects of advanced practice will differ according to the profession, specialty and place of care delivery (ICN, 2020) (RCN, 2024) (NMC, 2025). Planning care should be person-centred whatever aspect of treatment or care one is proposing to enable or deliver. This chapter will include a range of case studies to provide examples of care planning in advanced clinical practice in a variety of settings. Non-medical prescribing is now embedded within advanced clinical practice for many disciplines and is therefore included in the discussion within this chapter.

Learning outcomes

At the conclusion of this chapter, you will be able to:

- Critically examine the role of care planning in your area of work.
- Identify the range of skills required for successful care planning.
- Develop knowledge in enabling a holistic care planning approach.
- Develop skills in helping patients to set realistic goals.

Enabling concordance with healthy lifestyle choices, encouraging participation in appropriate screening programmes and achieving adherence to medication and treatment regimens is a goal to which all health care professionals should aspire. Person-centred care planning can provide a foundation on which to build therapeutic relationships, increase knowledge and develop the skills and competencies required by patients to

DOI: 10.4324/9781003609049-6

achieve their goals. There is increasing evidence that effective self-care interventions are as important as medical treatments in mitigating diseases (Ahmad Joshi 2023; Sanderson & White 2018; World Health Organisation 2024). The importance of the development of the ability to self-manage for the individual with a long-term condition is evident in the example of the patient with diabetes: It is estimated that in the UK a person with diabetes spends on average three hours per year in contact with practitioners (Diabetes UK 2022; National Diabetes Audit, 2024). The individual lives with, and manages, their condition within the society and culture that is shaped and informed by their own, family and peer knowledge, beliefs and skills, for an overwhelming majority of their life. The individual's ability to self-care can be influenced by positive interactions with health care professionals, who working with patients in a person-centred approach, can develop a care plan that takes into account the goals, values and preferences of the individual.

Background

Care planning is contextualised according to the specialty and environment in which the care delivery is planned and must be responsive to the needs of the individual (Royal College of Nursing, 2024). Using the example of care planning for patients with long-term conditions, there is a consensus that it is the process of collaborative and supportive care planning rather than the produced care plan which is important (Ajibade 2021; National Institute for Health and Care Excellence 2021; Roberts et al 2019). Many services and organisations will have templates and documents for written care plans and these vary in their aims and objectives. For the purposes of this chapter a care plan is simply defined as the product of a collaborative process. In the instance of a consultation for a minor ailment, this could be the outcome of a discussion between patient and health care provider that certain simple self-care measures be adopted and a review planned if there is no improvement in symptoms within a time frame. Alternatively, it could be a complex written document held by both the practitioner and the patient, detailing agreed specific goals and actions, some of which may be long-term goals such as weight loss, smoking cessation and/or concordance with complicated medication regimens.

Irrespective of the complexity and format of the plan, the defining characteristics of care planning should remain the same in order to achieve the anticipated outcomes. The plan must be:

- Holistic
- Person-centred; taking into account the person's values, goals and preferences
- Owned by the individual and be in a format which can be easily accessed and understood
- Goals must be realistic and achievable and have a time frame

The advanced practitioner will be required to draw on a range of skills and competencies to enable successful care planning (ICN, 2020). There are a range of tools in the form of competency frameworks which can help define standards, guide professional development and enable reflection on practice (Health Education England/HEE 2020; Keston & Beebe 2021; RPS 2021; RCGP 2015). The framework for

Advanced Clinical Practitioners working in primary care, developed by Skills for Health (Health Education England/HEE 2020), is aligned with the Multi-Disciplinary Framework for Advanced Clinical Practice in England (Health Education England/HEE 2020) and outlines four domains (Table 4.1). Underpinning these domains, thirteen capabilities are detailed outlining the skills, knowledge and behaviours required for nurses working at an advanced level.

The Royal Pharmaceutical Society (RPS) has developed a competency framework for all prescribers (RPS 2021). Many of the competencies in the RPS framework can be aligned with those in the Health Education England (Health Education England/HEE 2020) framework but are applied more specifically to the prescribing issues relevant in advanced clinical practice. The RPS provides a useful tool for those wishing to develop skills and review the need for continuing professional development in non-medical prescribing.

Prerequisites for planning care

The capabilities within Domain A 'Patient-centred collaborative working' (Table 4.2 , Capabilities in Domain A) will be used to focus a critical discussion in relation to care planning; it should be noted that the other domains in this framework also discuss relevant skills and competencies and are identified where applicable in the case studies. The practitioner must consider all the domains and capabilities when planning care with an individual. Good communication, necessary in all four domains, is essential in establishing a effective and meaningful relationship with patients and clients in order to negotiate a successful plan of care.

The following case study will be used to critically discuss elements of the communication and consultation domain and identify the relevance in care planning and ensuring effective practice.

Table 4.1 Domains A and B

Domain A	*Domain B*
Person-centred collaborative working	Assessment, investigations and diagnosis
Domain C	*Domain D*
Condition management, treatment and prevention	Leadership and management, education and research

(adapted from Health Education England/HEE 2020)

Table 4.2 Capabilities in Domain A

Capability 1. Communication and consultation skills
Capability 2. Practising holistically to personalise care and promote public and person health
Capability 3. Working with colleagues and in teams
Capability 4. Maintaining an ethical approach and fitness to practices

Source: Health Education England/HEE (2020).

Example 1

> S is a 49–year-old woman who has type 2 diabetes and hypertension; both diagnosed four years previously. S last attended a diabetes review at the practice ten months ago with different practitioner. At the last consultation a review date had been set for three months as her glycosylated haemoglobin (HbAlc) was considered high and a change in medication dosage made. At this consultation it was noted that S stated that she was taking her medication as prescribed. Since this time S has requested two repeat prescriptions (both issued for a one-month supply); the last request being four months previously. A review of the notes indicates that prior to the consultation ten months ago, S had only been prescribed a total of 90 days' supply in the previous 12 months. S had attended an appointment with a health care assistant who had taken blood tests and recorded Blood Pressure (BP) and weight two weeks ago. S is attending now for an annual review. Her test results show an increase in the HbAlc level and her BP remains elevated. S has lost 5kg in weight and her current BMI is 28. S received a letter explaining these results in the mail one week before she attends for her care planning consultation.

During the consultation, S reveals that she has not taken any of the prescribed medication. S requested the prescriptions and obtained the medication which is still in a cupboard at home. S states that this is because she has read the patient information leaflet and is scared of the side effects listed.
Domain A, Capability 1 (g) (Health Education England/HEE 2020) states that advanced practitioners should:

> Consult in a highly organised and structured way, with professional curiosity as required, whilst understanding the constraints of the time limited nature of consultations and ensure communication is safe and effective

Given the limited time usually available, the advanced practitioner must be able to quickly establish good communication and trust with an individual. In the example of S, where S is suffering from a long-term condition, the practitioner should review the history and be well informed about the condition to help gain trust of the individual. Knowledge of the patient also reassures the patient that the practitioner is interested and concerned. It is also essential that the practitioner gain the trust of others whom S may wish to include in planning her care, such as family members, who may have a considerable influence on S's future actions and behaviours. Mutual trust enables an environment in which the patient will feel able to accurately inform the practitioner about her concerns, identified problems, current lifestyle and medication use. S had stated at a previous consultation that she was taking the medication but a review of the records shows only a supply of 90 days' medications in a 12-month period. The practitioner needs to explore this anomaly with the patient to enable an understanding of why the patient is not taking the medicines as prescribed. In a context of mutual trust, where the practitioner shows real interest in the patient, this should be possible.
Domain A, Capability 1 (a) (Health Education England/HEE 2020) states that advanced practitioners should:

> Critically appraise communication strategies and be able to optimise communication approaches appropriately … e.g. frequently clarifying, paraphrasing and picking up on verbal cues

In order to elicit an accurate answer to these questions S must feel able to trust the practitioner. There are a wide range of verbal and non-verbal communication skills which can facilitate the establishment of trust and some of these are discussed later in this chapter. The practitioner must remain conscious of the social and cultural differences between patients when utilising these skills (3; Thompson 2010).
Domain A, Capability 1 (c) (Health Education England/HEE 2020) states that advanced practitioners should:

> Autonomously adapt verbal and non-verbal communication styles that are empathetic and responsive to people's communication and language needs, preferences and abilities (including levels of spoken English and health literacy)

An important part of establishing a successful therapeutic relationship with S will be establishing a no-blame culture to enable her to feel that she will not be judged or made to feel guilty about her lack of adherence to medication. It is also essential that the practitioner takes care not to create an environment which encourages patients to 'please' the practitioner by reporting complete concordance where none exists. It is important to approach S as more of an accountability partner, not a judge.
Domain A, Capability 1 (b) (Health Education England/HEE 2020) states that advanced practitioners should:

> Reflect on communication strategies and skilfully adapt those employed to ensure communication strategies foster an environment of person power

Creating a partnership with a patient and enabling shared decision making is viewed as essential in effecting improved health outcomes for patients in all aspects of care and treatment (Coulter et al 2015; NICE 2021). Patients present with a wide range of personal experiences, knowledge and beliefs and in order to influence any of these, the practitioner must first understand pre-existing conditions. In the first example, S presents as an individual with 'uncontrolled' long-term conditions according to the biochemical outcomes measures suggested in national guidance (NICE 2015). At this stage the practitioner does not have any knowledge of S's understanding of these diagnoses and implications for her health. The use of open questions will help to elicit a broad outline of the situation and the use of a closed question to focus in can be helpful. For example the open question:

> How do you think what you eat affects your diabetes?

Such a question could help the practitioner to gain an understanding of S's perceptions about her self-efficacy and self-knowledge as well as giving an understanding of her knowledge base. If the issue of food labelling comes up a further open question could be:

What do you think about the system of food labelling in the supermarkets? Have you had any information about food labels in the past?

Reflecting on the conversation can ensure that we have gained an accurate understanding of what we have been told and ensure that we don't allow any misconceptions to arise which may influence our future actions and negatively impact on the relationship with the patient.

S was noted to have lost weight at the review. She may raise this herself but the use of a focussed closed question can provide the practitioner with further understanding of any factors which may have affected this.

I notice that you have lost weight. Was this something you planned?

The outcome of the response to this question can help direct the practitioner to potential future education and support. If the weight loss is the result of a planned change in behaviour by S then acknowledgement of her success and further support to continue will be useful. If the weight loss is not planned and S is unaware of any changes which would have triggered this then this might indicate a need for a different plan of care entirely, including an assessment of risk for co-morbidities.

Activity 1

Think of a question that you use frequently in your area of work. Is it an open or closed question? Consider if this is the most appropriate type of question and consider what rationale you have for using it.

Active listening

The use of open or closed questions will help our understanding and enable the development of our relationship *only* if we are willing to listen to the answers. Active listening can be challenging, particularly in a situation where time is limited. The practitioner may be thinking ahead to the next question or may be distracted by interruptions. It is important that not only do we gain the information required, but that the patient feels that their words are being understood and valued in order to further develop the relationship of mutual trust. Active listening involves showing a response to what is being said, this can be verbal or non-verbal, but care must be taken to ensure that the focus remains with the speaker.

Verbal signals

The use of phrases such as 'go on' and 'I see' can ensure that you do not interrupt or draw attention away from what the patient is expressing but can indicate to the patient that you are interested and actively listening to their story. Tennant et al (2023) discuss the use of reflecting back and paraphrasing as tools in active listening to enhance empathy and trust. The use of these can also help us to prompt further information and to check the accuracy of our understanding.

Non-verbal signals

The practitioner must be aware of the non-verbal signals that are unconsciously sent. Body posture, head movements and eye contact all indicate to the person with whom we are interacting our level of interest in what they are saying and can also convey approval (or disapproval). The use of non-verbal signals can encourage the patient to continue talking and reveal more information or conversely can effectively draw a conversation to a premature end.

Monitor and reflect on your own emotional response

Domain A, Capability 4 (b) (Health Education England/HEE 2020) states that advanced practitioners should:

> Critically reflect on how own values, attitudes and beliefs might influence one's professional behaviour

Every practitioner works within a frame of reference influenced by previous experiences and personal beliefs. Understanding and acknowledging these beliefs and attitudes can enable the advanced practitioner to avoid adopting judgmental attitudes with patients who may choose a course of action which is not concordant with our view of the world. S has made a conscious decision not to take the medication and has not trusted others with this knowledge. It is essential that the practitioner responds in a non-judgmental way to S's revelation, taking an open approach that allows her to voice her concerns and doubts about any aspect of her care including the prescribing of medication. Any attempt to blame S will be detrimental to the relationship and is unlikely to result in increased adherence. The practitioner should use verbal and non-verbal skills to demonstrate an understanding of the complex reasons for her behaviour. Keeping the holistic approach in mind, practitioners should be prepared to provide patients with several treatment options including nonpharmacologic lifestyle modifications and different options for medications including different timings and routes of administration if available.

It is estimated that between 30% and 50% of medications prescribed for long-term conditions are not taken as prescribed (National Institute for Healthcare and Care Excellence, 2021). This non-adherence may be intentional or unintentional and is likely to be due to a multitude of factors. In S's example we clearly see a failure to agree on a shared plan of care initially – the practitioner issued a prescription for an increased dose of a medication which S had already made a decision not to take. In addition, there is no evidence of support for adherence to an agreed action. For instance, a plan to review after one month to check for side effects or to answer queries.

Activity 2

Think of a situation where a patient or client has not taken a medication as prescribed. Make a note of how you felt about this, how this influenced subsequent care and what actions you took. Consider what could have been done differently and how this would have influenced the outcomes.

The care planning process

'Care plans' have been employed in health care for many years but in the past they have often been led by clinicians, and the focus has been on the production of a written care plan to inform and direct a team of practitioners involved in the individual's care. In recent years there has been increasing evidence that shared decision making and emphasis on the process of care planning result in greater patient satisfaction and are more likely to achieve the goals identified in the final agreed care plan (Coulter et al 2022; National Institute for Healthcare and Care Excellence 2021; Roberts et al 2019).

The Year of Care Model outlines the following domains which must be shared and discussed in order to enable a holistic care planning consultation.

- Emotional
- Social
- Clinical
- Behavioural
- Knowledge and health beliefs

The model is predicated on active encouragement of the individual with the long-term condition to reflect on their 'story' and any questions or concerns they may have in advance of the shared meeting with the practitioner. The subsequent meeting requires equality between the practitioner and the patient with both having perspectives to share and discuss.

Timing

Domain A, Capability 2 (a) (Health Education England/HEE 2020) states that advanced practitioners should:

> Critically appraise the impact that a range of social, economic and environmental factors can have on health outcomes for people, and where applicable their family and carers

Example 2

> M is a 37-year-old Bengali man who attends a practice requesting help with stopping smoking. He has been smoking for 20 years and reports smoking 15 cigarettes a day. This has increased over the years from five cigarettes per day initially. The nurse calculates this as equivalent to 13 pack-years. M says he has to give up as he has been made redundant recently and financially he cannot afford to keep buying cigarettes. M's wife attends with him and says she is worried about his health as her father suffered from COPD and died aged 57 years.
>
> M attempted smoking cessation six months previously and used nicotine replacement patches. He stopped smoking completely for a period of two weeks and then restarted which M feels was due to stress at work.

The process of any change in behaviour begins with the identification of a need or desire to change. The identification may arise from within an individual, be prompted by a person with significant influence such as a close friend or colleague or may come from a health care worker. In the case study given, M indicates that the trigger for his deciding to attempt behaviour change is the financial cost of continuing to smoke. Whatever the trigger, any attempt to coerce or persuade an individual to change behaviour is unlikely to succeed and may in fact damage the therapeutic relationship. The stages of change theoretical model developed by Prochaska and DiClemente (1986) outlined five stages of change. These are:

Precontemplation – the patient is not contemplating any change within the next six months
Contemplation – there is an intention to change within the next few months
Preparation – the patient is making plans to change in the near future
Action – the stage during which the patient is making specific behavioural changes
Maintenance – this period is estimated to last from six months to five years.

This was later updated to include a sixth stage – termination – a term used to describe a stage whereby the individual no longer has any desire to relapse regardless of any mitigating factors. Using this trans-theoretical model can help us understand M's progress in his attempts to stop smoking; his relapse and preparation to try again. It can also help us to understand the need for support during the action and maintenance stages.

Domain B, Capability 5 (b) (Health Education England/HEE 2020) states that advanced practitioners should:

> Use active listening skills and open questions to effectively engage and facilitate shared agenda setting

Motivational interviewing (MI) is an approach which can be used to explore factors which could motivate and identify any potential barriers to change with an individual. MI aims to utilise the patient's own goals and system of values to stimulate a desired change in behaviour. A basic tenet of the approach is that the motivation to change is elicited from the patient and not imposed; the skilled motivational interviewer will gain an understanding of the individual's motivating factors and reinforce these whilst challenging any barriers which are elicited. In M's case, this could involve discussing the financial cost of smoking and calculating a monthly or annual figure to reinforce the benefit to the family finances. The use of support and reinforcement to empower the individual to change is central to the approach and the patient's belief in their self-efficacy is essential.

The four key stages of MI can be viewed as:

(1) **Engaging.** Establishing a working relationship, using open questions and finding out about M's perspective regarding his smoking habit.
(2) **Focussing.** Encouraging M to identify and focus on his agenda, ensuring this is achievable for him.

(3) **Evoking.** Encourage M to identify his own motivations for change. This may include actively listening to why he should not stop smoking, enabling M to look at both sides of the argument whilst keeping a focus on his strengths and reasons for changing.
(4) **Planning.** This must be a collaborative process; M should be encouraged to identify his own solutions where possible, although the practitioner should be prepared to offer information and advice if invited by M. For example, discuss various reasons for relapses or barriers to the goal, and identify realistic, positive coping mechanisms to avoid relapse or barriers; in M's case, stress at work.

A Cochrane review of randomised controlled trials using MI in smoking cessation was cautious in its analysis of effectiveness due to variations in study quality but concluded that it may help smokers to quit (Lai et al. 2010).

Eliciting
Example 3

> A need was identified to increase the uptake of childhood vaccinations in a multicultural inner-city area, as levels of uptake were insufficient to assume herd immunity. It was assumed that the controversy regarding MMR vaccination was largely responsible for a decline in confidence in the programme and the low uptake of vaccination. A network of four GP practices planned an event incorporating entertainment activities for children, experienced nurses to discuss immunisation with parents, and to offer immunisation if required. A presentation was prepared on MMR vaccination and delivered twice during the day. The expert delivering the presentation was also available for discussion with parents. All parents of children who had not completed a full vaccination schedule received an invitation to the day.

The issue of assessing need in an individual is discussed earlier in this chapter. The practitioner may also be called upon to assess need and plan care for a group of individuals. In this case study the need was identified using data which showed levels of uptake insufficient to assume herd immunity. An assumption was made that the controversy regarding MMR vaccination was largely responsible for a decline in confidence in the programme and the low uptake of vaccination. This assessment was based on anecdotal evidence from practitioners in the area and discussions in the media.

The MMR expert delivered the presentation which was well received. During discussions with parents, the expert received several queries about polio vaccination from parents who had recently emigrated from eastern Europe. It emerged that the live polio vaccine was being used in some countries and concerns had been raised about polio vaccine-related morbidity.

In this example, the practitioners had made assumptions about the cause of low uptake for vaccination which prove to be, at least partially, inaccurate. We must take care to ensure that our assessment is thorough and encompasses a wider evidence base than can be gained from personal experiences. In this situation the influences gained from peers within a cultural group had caused parents to make a decision not to vaccinate their children. The need for use of public health information and epidemiological data is identified in Domain D of the framework (Health Education England/HEE 2020)

Enabling
Example 4

> A, a 35-year-old woman attended a family planning clinic requesting the combined oral contraceptive pill (COC) as she had previously been prescribed this elsewhere. The practitioner undertook a full assessment encompassing previous medical history, a gynaecological history, family history, BP, weight, BMI and smoking history. The practitioner used the information gained to assess the suitability of this method for A and concluded that in line with current guidance the method was contraindicated.
>
> Domain B, Capability 5 (e) (Health Education England/HEE 2020) states that advanced practitioners should:
>
> 'Be able to undertake general history-taking, and focussed history taking to elicit and assess 'red flags'

This example requires a careful discussion with A so that A will understand why the method is contraindicated. Initially the practitioner must assess how much A understands about the drug and possible risk and benefits. It is also important to gain an understanding of A's previous experiences with contraception and her need for this contraceptive therapy. Open questioning around previous discussions with practitioners would provide insight into A's knowledge in this area.

Domain B, Capability 5 (i) (Health Education England/HEE 2020) states that advanced practitioners should:

> Deliver diagnosis and test/investigation results, (including bad news) sensitively and appropriately in line with local or national guidance …
>
> Domain B, Capability 5 (i) (Health Education England/HEE 2020)

The practitioner informs A that the method is contraindicated, and she must stop taking it. A is very upset. She has had problems in the past with dysmenorrhea which was relieved by the COC. A feels that this issue was not raised by her previousGeneral Practitioner GP (Family Practitioner/Doctor). The practitioner feels defensive, but is sure that she is right, and that to prescribe the COC would not be in the patient's interests. A immediately leaves the consultation feeling frustrated that she cannot obtain the treatment she wishes to have.

This outcome clearly demonstrates the poor outcomes which can be expected when the practitioner fails to gain an understanding of A's perceived 'need' for the COC. In this case study, had the practitioner approached the situation more sensitively and provided options for other more suitable methods of contraception, the outcome may have been very different. A would have been enabled to make a decision regarding the form of contraception. In this situation, the practitioner must also watch for A's emotional response. Defensive behaviour is likely to result in the rapid deterioration of a therapeutic relationship.

> **Activity 3**
> Using the above case study, consider how the practitioner could have approached this situation and what techniques could have been used to improve the outcome so that A could have been enabled to make an appropriate decision regarding contraception.

Providing
Example 5

> Mr K is a 65-year-old man who was diagnosed with type 2 diabetes two years ago. He attended two weeks ago and had blood and urine tests, BP, weight and a foot check. At this consultation the practitioner discussed Mr K's lifestyle in terms of diet and exercise patterns and had referred Mr K to a local exercise scheme. Mr K had received the results of the assessment via text message a few days before the care planning consultation. The results show that Mr K has gained weight and his HbA1c has increased over the past 6 months.

Domain A, Capability 2 (i) (Health Education England/HEE 2020) states that advanced practitioners should:

> Develop and promote shared management/personalised care/support plans with people individualised to meet their needs in partnership…

The Year of Care model being used in this context provides Mr K with information about the results of parameters used to determine the current state of control of his diabetes. Traditionally the practitioner would hold this information and would 'give' whatever the practitioner felt appropriate to the patient when the patient attended the consultation. The use of a traditional medical model ensures that the clinician remains in control, holding the information about test results, and leads to a disempowered patient who has insufficient information to make informed decisions. Receiving the information in advance also allows Mr K time to reflect on the results and any possible contributing factors.

> The practitioner asks Mr K if there are any questions he has about the results letter.

Domain B, Capability 5 (c) (Health Education England/HEE 2020) states that advanced practitioners should:

> Explore and appraise peoples' ideas, concerns and expectations about their symptom and condition and whether these may act as a driver or form a barrier

Mr K asks some questions about the exact nature of the kidney tests and he demonstrates a good understanding of the answers. The practitioner must ensure that an individual has a good understanding of any relevant literature included in the results text message. The use of written literature must be approached sensitively. An individual may find it difficult to acknowledge that they cannot read or write and in some spoken languages there may not be a written language.

The practitioner asks Mr K whether he feels any of the results should be improved.

Asking Mr K to identify his priorities will help to ensure that any of his concerns are addressed first and enables the practitioner to develop an understanding of what goals Mr K might wish to address. The results of an ensuing discussion will allow the practitioner to identify key areas of educational need and a plan can begin to be developed between the practitioner and the patient.

The consultation must be adapted to suit not only an individual's communication and learning preferences but must also be culturally relevant and sensitive.

Negotiating

Example 6

> L is a 44-year-old Caucasian woman who was diagnosed with hypertension four years ago. L works full time in a career which requires extensive travelling, staying in hotels and entertaining clients.. L was noted as having a BMI of 30 at diagnosis and has since gained a further 7 kg. Her BMI is now 36. L is unhappy about this weight gain. L attends her local GP practice requesting medication to aid weight loss and after discussing a range of options, a plan is agreed to a trial of a Glucagon-like peptide 1 (GLP-1) medication. Currently, in England, this medication would not be available to L on an NHS prescription, adding an extra layer of financial complexity.
>
> Domain A, Capability 2 (h) (Health Education England/HEE 2020) states that advanced practitioners should:
>
> 'Engage people in shared decision making about their care by .... Exploring with them the risks and benefits of each available option, discussing implications, how it related to them and promoting their understanding as much as possible'

Negotiation requires both parties to understand and share a common goal. If the practitioner identifies a need for weight loss but the patient does not view this goal as a priority it is unlikely that any change in behaviour leading to weight loss will occur. In the case of L, she had already identified the goal of weight loss and declared herself ready to address the weight gain, and is prepared to spend a considerable amount of money to achieve this goal. There will be many contributing elements to the care plan including education and support for learning in knowledge of food types and portion sizes and support for increasing physical activity (perhaps referral to exercise schemes), all of which will require negotiation. A plan may be agreed on for L to start walking to work in the morning but if, at review, this goal has not been achieved then clearly a change of approach or goal is required. Perhaps the goal was too ambitious – the walk too far or time consuming; the route may be unpleasant or considered unsafe to walk. Using the skills discussed earlier in the chapter to elicit the barriers can aid in the development of realistic goals.

L has requested medication to help her weight loss and the plan of care agreed includes the use of this drug. The practitioner, using national guidance, discusses target weight loss with L and agrees on an initial review date to check concordance with medication and injection technique and to address any potential side effects.

Domain C, Capability 8 (f) (Health Education England/HEE 2020) states that advanced practitioners should:

> 'Evaluate outcomes of care against existing standards and patient outcomes and manage/adjust plans appropriately in line with best available evidence'
>
> L attends for an efficacy review after three months and has lost 2kg, which is half the agreed goal st at the care planning consultation. L is disappointed, stating that she feels she had lost more than this but last week she had a family crisis and had less time to plan and prepare meals and was relying on takeaways.

The practitioner must continually evaluate an individual's motivation, plan tolerance (i.e. medications, time to implement plan and stressors) and readiness to change. It would be appropriate to reflect back to L the situation and directly challenge her readiness for change. The practitioner might say something like:

> So things have been stressful and you have not really been able to keep to the plan. Is this something that is now resolved?

Coaching
Example 6 continued

> L reveals that her younger brother had peritonitis and was very ill. He is now making a good recovery. L says that this was a one-off situation; that everything is resolved and she is ready to try again.

The practitioner will empathise with an obviously stressful and traumatic situation. The coaching function describes the use of reminding, support and encouraging. The practitioner can use the weight loss, although small, to encourage L and discuss the fact that she had effectively changed her behaviour for a period, indicating her efficacy to do so again. The use of this support for self-efficacy is consistent with the principles in MI discussed previously. The opportunity should be taken to assess the need for further educational needs identified by L or any barrier encountered. The care plan should be reviewed in terms of the actions and goals and agreed on in the light of the previous experiences. Another review date should be identified.

Domain C, Capability 8 (i) (Health Education England/HEE 2020) states that advanced practitioners should:

> Suggest a variety of follow-up arrangements that are safe and appropriate, whilst also enhancing the person's autonomy

If the situation affecting L is ongoing, she must be given the opportunity and space to decide that this is not the right time to engage and a plan could simply be that a review will take place after a period of time and another assessment made of her readiness to change. It is important to remember the earlier discussion about emotional response in this situation. The practitioner may feel that there has been a significant investment in time, financial resources in medication costs and effort and feel frustrated at the lack of change. However, the practitioner must accept that there may be other external influences which bring a stronger imperative and therefore the 'investment' will not yield the desired response at this particular time.

Conclusion

This chapter has used the framework for Advanced Clinical Practitioners working in primary care, to critically examine many of the skills and competencies required in planning care with patients and has considered the use of skills identified in MI. There are many other theoretical models and frameworks which practitioners will find contribute to the development of effective care planning. Care planning must be a flexible process which accounts for each patient who, as a unique individual, will require a different approach and have a different set of goals. Arguably the most important element of the care plan is that both the individual and health care professional are actively working towards common goals. The use of a care planning process to successfully promote health and well-being is a challenging role, and in some areas of practice this will involve a team approach contributed to by many practitioners, whereas in others it may only involve an individual practitioner. However, whatever the setting, the approach must always remain centred around the person.

References

Ahmad, F and Joshi, S H (2023) *Self-Care Practices and Their Role in the Control of Diabetes: A Narrative Review*. India: Cureus.

Ajibade, B (2021) *Assessing the patient's needs and planning effective care. British Journal of Nursing* 30 (20): pp 1166–1171

Coulter, A, Collins, A, Edwards, A, Entwistle, V, Finnikin, S, Jospeh-Williams, N, Thomas, V and Thomson, R (2022) *Implementing Shared Decision Making in the UK*: Progress 2017-2022 EPub 2022 May 21.

Coulter, A, Entwistle, V A, Eccles, A, Ryan, S, Sheppherd, S and Perera, R (2015) *Personalised care planning for adults with chronic or long-term health conditions: Review. Cochrane Database of Systematic Reviews* \ 3: CD010523. doi: 10.1002/14651858.CD010523.pub2.

Diabetes UK (2022) *Easing the Burden for People with Diabetes*. Diabetes UK.

Health Education England, NHS England & Skills for Health (HEE, 2020) *Core Capabilities Framework for Advanced Clinical Practice (Nurses) Working in General Practice/Primary Care in England*. Skills for Health.

International Council of Nurses (ICN 2020) *Guidelines on Advanced Practice Nursing*. Switzerland: ICN.

Keston, K S and Beebe, S L (2021) *Competency Frameworks for nurse practitioner residency and fellowship programs: Comparison, analysis and recommendations*. American Association of Nurse Practitioners. 34 (1): 160–168.

Lai, D T, Cahill, K, Qin, Y and Tang, J L (2010) Motivational interviewing for smoking cessation. *Cochrane Database Systematic Review* 2010 Jan 20th (). CD006936. https://pubmed.ncbi.nlm.nih.gov/20091612/ (Accessed 05/06/226).

National Diabetes Audit (2024) *Quarterly Report April to September 2024*. NHS Digital. https://digital.nhs.uk/data-and-information/publications/statistical/national-diabetes-audit (Accessed 05/06/26).

National Institute for Health and Care Excellence (2015) *Type 2 Diabetes in Adults: Management: Updated 29th June 2022*. London: National Institute for Health and Care Excellence.

National Institute for Health and Care Excellence (2021) *Shared decision making (NG197)*. London: National Institute for Health and Care Excellence.

Nursing and Midwifery Council (NMC, 2025) *Principles for Advanced Practice*. London: NMC.

Prochaska, J. O. and DiClemente, C. C. (1986) Toward a comprehensive model of change. In: W.R. Miller and N. Heather, (Eds). *Treating Addictive Behaviours: Processes of Change*. New York: Plenum Press.

Roberts, S, Eaton, S, Finch, T, Lewis-Barned, N, Lhussier, M, Oliver, L, Rapley, T and Temple-Scott, D (2019) *The Year of Care Approach; Developing and Model and Delivery Programme for Care and Support Planning in Long Term Conditions within General Practice*. UK: BMC Family Practice.

Royal College of General Practitioners (2015) *General Practice Nurse Competencies*. London: RCGP Publishing.

Royal College of Nursing (RCN, 2024) *RCN Professional Development Framework – Levels of Nursing, Advanced Level Nursing*. London: RCN Publishing.

Royal Pharmaceutical Society (2021) *A Competency Framework for All Prescribers*. London: RPS.

Sanderson, J and White, J (2018) *Making the case for a personalised approach*. NHS England.

Taylan, C and Weber, L T (2023) *"Don't let me be misunderstood": communication with patients from a different cultural background* Paediatric Nephrology 38 (3): pp 643–649. https://pubmed.ncbi.nlm.nih.gov/35930048/ (Accessed 05/06/26).

Tennant, K., Long, A. and Toney-Butler, T. (2023) Active Listening. National Library of Medicine. September, 2023. www.ncbi.nlm.nih.gov/books/NBK442015/ (Accessed 05/06/26)

Thompson, K. (2010) Working with individuals and groups: Creating and strengthening relationships. In: C. L. Cox and M. C. Hill, (Eds). *Professional Issues in Primary Care Nursing*. Oxford: Wiley-Blackwell.

World Health Organisation (2024) *Self-care for health and well-being* www.who.int/news-room/fact-sheets/detail/self-care-health-interventions (accessed 2nd July 2025).

PART 2

Management

CHAPTER 5

Management theory

Marie C. Hill

Introduction

The role of the Registered Nurse (RN) and Allied Health Professional (AHP) has changed significantly in the United Kingdom (UK) since the 1990s, particularly in the context of advanced clinical practice. These role changes have occurred for a number of reasons, due to the complexity of an increasing ageing population health workforce shortages and escalating health costs (Salsberg and Quigley, 2017). With these challenges to health care systems, there have been ongoing debates how to meet health care needs effectively (Evans et al, 2020). In the UK, this has led to an increase in services from the acute sector to primary care and with this a need to examine who provides these increased services. The recently published *Fit for the Future: 10 Year Health Plan for England* has further endorsed the shift in how the NHS works with:

- More care available in the community setting
- Availability and use of new technologies
- Greater emphasis on preventative strategies (NHS, 2025)

This has led to new opportunities for RNs and AHPs to take on roles previously within the domain of a general practitioner (GP), particularly advanced clinical practice. It can be argued that these changes not only promote these professional groups but highlight the career opportunities and different pathways and choices that are now available in advanced clinical practice. It has been contended that advanced clinical practitioners (ACPs) are in an ideal position to take on future managers' roles in healthcare (Addison and Scott, 2025).

The aim of this chapter is to explore management in terms of definition and theories of management including their influence on today's health care organisations.

Learning outcomes

At the conclusion of this chapter, you will be able to:

DOI: 10.4324/9781003609049-8

- Explore the various definitions of management and distinguish management from administration
- Understand how management theory has evolved and developed
- Critically appraise the diverse role of the manager
- Examine some of the strategies that managers use

Background

What is management?

The distinction between leadership and management has long been debated. There is ambiguity about the boundaries between leadership and management roles, with these terms used interchangeably, especially in healthcare (Addison and Scott, 2025). This has led some to contend that being a manager and a leader at the same time is a viable concept (Huston, 2022). It has been asserted that a good manager should embody both leadership and management qualities to handle their role effectively (Addison and Scott, 2025). However, it is not the intention of this chapter to delineate between leadership and management, as firstly leadership will be explored in detail later in this book and secondly, the focus of this chapter is on management with particular emphasis on advanced clinical practice.

Management has been defined as: the act or art of managing: the conducting or supervising of something (such as a business) (Merriam Webster Dictionary, 2025). Management in healthcare has been described as consisting of six critical tasks, namely: planning; allocating resources; co-ordinating the work of others; motivating staff; monitoring output and taking responsibility for the process that underpins the delivery of care (Jones et al, 2022).

In Drucker's (1968) book *The Practice of Management*, it was advocated that questioning the exact functions of a manager's role would shed light on a more precise definition of their role and responsibilities. Mintzberg's (1973) definition of the role of manager contrasts in some respects to that of Handy's, who identified the role of a manager as one of involving leadership, administration and resolving (Handy, 1999). Mintzberg viewed that there were three distinct categories to a manager's role:

- Interpersonal
- Leader and liaison
- Information, which is monitor, disseminator spokesman and finally, decisional roles which are entrepreneur, resource allocator and negotiator

(Jones and Jenkins, 2006)

Therefore, the administrative role is but one of the many roles that a manager holds and is not an exclusive role. In appraising organisational effectiveness of a manager, it was viewed that this flowed from the interaction and relationship between several factors, which were described as the 7-S framework (Mintzberg et al, 1995). The constituent parts of the 7-S framework were:

Systems

These relate to the formal and informal procedures of the organisation. For example, budgeting and training.

Style

This relates to how power within a team or organisation is managed. This could be in relation to how managers spend their time and could be symbolic in how the team is perceived as managing their time.

Staff

This is two-tiered. Firstly, it relates to appraisal systems and training initiatives and/or programmes with the latter being formal rather than informal training. For example, attendance at a Higher Education Institution for an academic programme (e.g., a Masters in Business Administration or a Postgraduate Diploma in Primary Care Practice Nursing).

Skills

This relates to current skills and skills that need to be acquired. The latter being identified as new roles that change and evolve within an organisation.

Strategy

This is a key function of any organisation and relates to how the organisation needs to change, be responsive to and adapt its functions in response to external forces. For example, a Health Maintenance Organisation (HMO) in the United States of America (USA) or a National Health Service (NHS) Trust (UK) expanding services in the provision of diabetes mellitus specialist nurses due to the higher prevalence and incidence of this long-term condition compared to the national average.

Structure

This is how the tasks are delegated within an organisation or team. There is a very strong association here with the 'Skills' function.

Superordinate goals

It is important for any manager, particularly in a health care environment, to understand factors that can influence their team's or organisation's effectiveness.

Activity 1

Consider the Mintzberg et al. 7-S framework and appraise the following:

How does this framework fit into the team that you manage or would like to manage?
What factors are strengths in the team?
What are the areas for improvement?
How would you improve these?
Can you identify any barriers to change?

The evolution of management theory

The role of the manager is diverse. How has management theory evolved to enable us to understand management in its present-day format? Management theory, as with the definition of management, has not been static and the theory itself has been responsive to change due to societal and organisational structure. The birth and development of management theory has been influenced by other disciplines such as business; psychology; sociology and anthropology (Marquis and Huston, 2009). The following will be an overview of the development and changes in management theory with examples from contributors to management theory and how these changes have influenced management in organisations, beginning with classical theories to modern-day approaches to management theory.

It was the beginning of the 20th century in 1925 when Henri Fayol first explored a definition of management and the general principles of management (Cole and Kelly, 2020). His experiences as a mining engineer and latterly as the managing director of the same company led him to publish his work on management and the identification of management functions, namely: planning; organisation; command; coordination and control (Huston, 2022). These management functions are considered to be the 'foundation stones of modern management' (Burtonshaw-Gunn, 2008:132). It was Luther Gulick in 1937 who expanded on Fayol's functions as identified by the following mnemonic – POSDCORB

- Planning
- Organising
- Staffing
- Directing
- Coordinating
- Reporting
- Budgeting

(Srinu, 2023)

In essence, Fayol and Gulick laid the framework for the organisation of both work and people.

This formal structure of management theory became known as the Classical Theory of Management. Unlike Fayol and Gulick, Elton Mayo viewed individuals within organisations as key to achieving organisational effectiveness (Cole and Kelly, 2020). He was the first of a number of theorists (e.g., Maslow, MacGregor, Argyris, Likert and Herzberg) to form what is termed the Human Relations and Social Psychological School of management theory (Cole and Kelly, 2020). Mayo's research was undertaken over a five-year period at the Hawthorne works of the Western Electric Company in Chicago. Overall, the research (i.e., from 1924 to 1936 in five distinct stages) revealed that productivity increased even though improvements in working conditions were taken away and productivity results were similar to the control group who did not have these improvements taken away. It was contended that this *Hawthorne effect* indicated that people respond to being studied and attempt to increase the behaviour they feel will continue to warrant attention (Huston, 2022). However, there have been critiques of the Hawthorne research. In a systematic review of 19 studies examining the *Hawthorne effect*, the overall conclusion was that while consequences of research participation for behaviours being investigated do exist, little can be securely known about the conditions under which they operate, their mechanisms of effects or their magnitudes. Therefore, it has been recommended that new concepts are needed to guide empirical studies (McCambridge et al, 2014).

Mayo and his colleagues influenced Abraham Maslow and his research into human motivation, which made a significant impact on developments in management theory during the 1950s–1960s (Cole and Kelly, 2020). Maslow proposed that the majority of people are motivated by the desire to satisfy specific groups of needs. His theory (i.e., the hierarchy-of-needs theory) is represented by the figure of a pyramid with the more basic 'Psychological needs' forming the base of the structure and the most desirable or highest needs in this figure at the top of the pyramid, 'Self-actualisation'. Refer to Figure 5.1. Maslow's needs were as follows:

- Physiological needs
- Safety needs
- Love needs
- Esteem need
- Self-actualisation needs

(Cole and Kelly, 2020)

Although Maslow's work has been highly influential in understanding human motivation, it has been criticised as being too simplistic in assuming that individuals' needs are standardised and for the fact that the theory heavily relied on Maslow's personal observations and clinical experiences (Saif, 2024). Furthermore, his motivational theory does not consider cultural and individual differences (Marriner Tomey, 2000). There are a number of other motivational theories, such as Roethlisberger and Dickson; Hezberg;

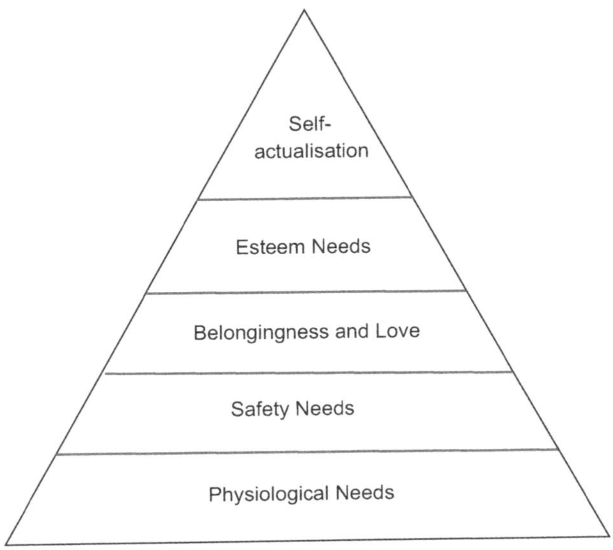

Figure 5.1 Maslow's Hierarchy of Needs

McClelland and Ardrey. Readers are referred to Handy's (1999) book *Understanding Organisations* for further information.

Another influence in management theory emerged around the same period as Fayol. Max Weber, a sociologist and known as the father of organisational theory, was interested in why individuals in organisations obeyed those in authority (Huston, 2022). Weber identified three types of legitimate authority that are: traditional; charismatic and rational-legal authority (Weber, 1947). It was the publication of Weber's translated text from *The Theory of Economic and Social Organisation* in 1947 where the term 'bureaucracy' was used to describe a rational form of organisation (Cole and Kelly, 2020). Whilst Weber identified the main features of a bureaucracy as in essence bound by rules and regulations, there have been critics of this form of management which is referred to as 'the dysfunctional consequences of bureaucracy' (Carnell, 2007:130). Some of these consequences have been summarised as an over-reliance on rules and structure, relationships are predictable based on the role of the individual leading to rigid conformity to the rules and consequently that change is difficult due to adherence to rigid rules and regulations (Cole and Kelly, 2020). Regardless of Weber's detractors, and that his work did not consider the complexity of managing organisations in the 21st century, his influence on management theory and administration have been influential (Langer, 2022).

Following on from the Human Relations and Social Psychological School of management theory, another school of thought began to emerge in the late 1960s. Douglas MacGregor proposed that managerial attitudes towards employees are closely linked to employee satisfaction (MacGregor, 1960). He categorised these attitudes into two distinct frameworks: *Theory X* and *Theory Y.*

According to *Theory X*, managers perceive employees as inherently lazy, requiring constant supervision and direction. In contrast, *Theory Y* suggests that managers view employees as intrinsically motivated, enjoying their work and striving to achieve both personal and organisational goals (Huston, 2022). Support for MacGregor's perspective has emerged over time, with scholars such as Argyris (2017) arguing that excessive managerial control can lead to employee passivity and discouragement. Despite limited empirical validation MacGregor's theories have significantly shaped management practices for nearly six decades (Prottas and Nummelin, 2018).

From the open systems theory of management emerged the contingency approach to management.

The latter theory viewed that a mixture of management theories could be adapted to an organisation. Handy in *Understanding Organisations* argued against a 'universal formula' or one size that fits all theory (Handy, 1999:181). However, he noted that 'most modern theories of organisations are increasingly persuaded of the wisdom ... of the match of people to systems, to task and environment, of inter-relations between all four' (Handy, 1999:181).

Activity 2

Reflect on your team and/or organisation. Considering the theories of management that you have read about.

What is the focus of your organisation? Does the team or organisation focus on task?
Is the team or organisation people focused or is it responsive to environmental change (i.e., proactive or reactive)? Do you consider that there are other factors that underpin the management of your team or organisation?

List these factors and consider what the drivers and barriers to change are in relation to your team or organisation.

This section on management theory introduces some of the influences on today's organisations. How does management theory influence an ACP in an ever-changing health care environment? To mirror Handy's words, the emphasis surely must be on the match of the individual, their role or task, the environment and the interconnection amongst these factors. How does an ACP deal with the complex interrelations on a team basis or in the wider organisation to meet the needs of the team and ultimately the organisation?

Managing people

Managing teams can be complex and challenging, as teams are not homogenous because of the diversity of each team. Therefore, an ACP must acknowledge and work with each individual within their team in order to have a functional team. Hunt (1992) asserts that managers must have a mixture of skills and competencies to manage effectively. These skills and competencies are having interpersonal, knowledge and visionary skills. Yukl and Gardener (2020) have examined a number of characteristics that effective managers possess, namely:

- Take advantage of reactive activities (i.e. they problem solve, influence others)
- Develop a large network of contacts
- Identify relationships between problems
- Learn from surprises and failures. In this instance the manager is open to suggestions and change
- Are willing to experiment and take chances
- Prioritise problems. This involves examining a trivial problem from e a major problem
- Are politically astute. This requires skill in understanding the organisation, its key people and how it works. For example, knowing who has influence in the organisation
- Allow time for reflective planning.

The effective manager needs time to consider plans and how to implement them. Some managers will be creative in how they set aside 'thinking time' to enable them to consider different options to a solution and how best to approach such a solution. There are many reflective models that can be utilised (e.g., Gibbs, 1988; Schon, 1987; Boud et al., 1985). Whatever reflective model is used will depend on a manager's previous experience of using a reflective model. Nevertheless, the use of a reflective model will allow and enable the manager to consider a situation or a problem that they wish to gain further insight into and/or to resolve.

Clearly, not all managers will have these skill sets. This raises the importance of health care organisations supporting and developing their managers to their potential. Iles (2006) has described three fundamental rules that a manager needs to follow to manage people effectively. These rules are:

- Clarity on what is expected of the team member to achieve
- Ensuring that the team member has the skills to achieve what is expected to be achieved
- Providing feedback on performance

These three rules are now explored in more detail.

Clarity on what is expected of the team member to achieve

This may seem obvious, but the question must be raised: do all managers engage with their team to ensure that they fully understand what they are expected to achieve in their role? Job descriptions are helpful, but in times of organisational growth and even uncertainty, there can be a lack of understanding by a manager on what they expect their team members to achieve. The role of the manager, therefore, is crucial in defining role expectations and especially how this is communicated to their team. It has been argued that assertive and effective communication is the key to relaying information to others (i.e., the information being relayed is clear and concise) (LaGanga, 2019; Sully and Dallas, 2005). It is for the manager to initiate the regularity of meetings with their team members.

Ensuring that the team member has the skills to achieve what is expected to be achieved

An important point for any manager (i.e., whether they have been promoted in their current organisation or moved to a new organisation) is to individually meet their team members and ascertain what skills they have or indeed do not possess to be able to meet the organisation's objectives. The role of the manager and the skills that are required are complex. Such skills include the acquisition of personal skills (i.e., Developing self-awareness; Managing stress and well-being; Solving problems analytically and creatively), interpersonal skills (i.e., Building relationship by communicating supportively; Gaining power and influence; Motivating performance; Negotiating and resolving conflict) and group skills (i.e., Empowering and engaging others; Building effective teams and teamwork; Leading positive change) (Whetten and Cameron, 2024).

For example, an ACP who has a partnership in a general practice is keen to increase patient access to services and to reduce waiting times. This ACP would need to ascertain the level of skills and competence that the other members of the team have. Following meetings with individual team members and the whole team, it was identified that there was a need for advanced physical assessment training to be undertaken by one member of the nursing team in order to meet the objectives of increasing services and reducing waiting times. Through the conduction of a needs assessment, other needs for education and training may be identified so that the RN has a range of skills and competence to assess, manage and treat clients as necessary. The ACP who manages this team would have to consider how they supervise and support the team member whilst they are undertaking education and training. Key for the ACP would be to ensure that the clinical practice of the RN, in this instance, is competent, safe and underpinned with a robust evidence base. What may be the most challenging aspect for the ACP in this instance is that their enthusiasm to implement change must take into consideration the support needs of the team member in terms of supervision and mentor support.

Providing feedback on performance

Following on from these two fundamental rules as identified by Iles (2006), the final rule is providing feedback on the team member's performance. This is essential for any manager in order for individuals to progress and achieve their set goals. Annual and mid-term appraisals are a way in which one-to-one feedback on a team member's performance can be given. Indeed, the developing of what is called a continuous feedback programme, feedback-friendly culture or positive feedback environment has often been advocated (Mertens et al, 2021). Therefore, providing feedback needs to be flexible in how this is undertaken, and a manager may need to provide this feedback on a regular basis, especially if they are supervising clinical practice. It can be seen from this example that an effective manager must be in tune with their team's needs and provide feedback when it is necessary. This will not only enhance their relationship with the team but promote a functioning team with competent members who are supported and recognised for their contribution to the organisation (Anderson, 2018; Sully and Dallas, 2005).

Activity 3

You are an ACP who needs to implement a change to service provision within your team. The Chief Executive Officer (CEO) within your organisation has made it clear that an increase in your service provision needs to be 'immediate'. You know the abilities of your team and that any increase in additional services will need training and supervision over at least a period of six months. The other solution would be to recruit, but the CEO has not contemplated this and has informed you that 'you must use the skills of your existing team, as we have no money to recruit new staff'.

You are one of the 'rising stars' of your organisation. You are considering applying for a senior management post, which you know will be advertised in the next three months. Therefore, it is essential that you and the team perform well. However, you consider that the CEO's time frame is unrealistic.

You do not wish to jeopardise your standing in the organisation because of the forthcoming senior management post. You know there is a solution to this and have the weekend to prepare for your meeting with the CEO on Monday morning. How would you approach this problem? You realise that change is inevitable and therefore, you must develop a business plan that is acceptable to the CEO but also to your team. How will you address this to both the CEO and your team?

Conclusion

Today's ACP who additionally may have a managerial role must possess a range of skills that not only include excellent interpersonal skills, but also a critical understanding and indeed an ability to apply management theory. This is key to the success of the manager's role in terms of dealing with day-to-day operational issues. As identified by Handy (1999), there is no universal management theory that meets every organisation's managerial needs, as organisations are not homogenous entities. What is important though is that a manager understands their team and individuals' roles. Ultimately, this may be easier for managers of a small team (e.g., less than ten) in comparison to a team larger than this. However, this will depend on the skills of the manager in how they 'ring fence' time for their team members and, notwithstanding, how they manage their own time.

What is not made explicit to the manager working at an advanced clinical practice level is how they deal with day-to-day operational issues such as negotiation, influencing, managing change and conflict resolution. The following chapters of this book will illustrate for you how to address these issues.

Ultimately, management is giving others the tools and resources to deliver, which is succinctly described by Seden and Reynolds (2003:5) as 'Giving people the ability to do the job that's in front of them'.

References

Addison, E. and Scott, V. J. (2025). Advanced clinical practitioners' untapped potential to become managers. *British Journal of Nursing*, 34(3), pp.174–183.

Anderson, C. (2018). Exploring the role of advanced nurse practitioners in leadership. *Nursing Standard*. doi: 10.7748/ ns.2018.e11044

Argyris, C. (2017). *Integrating the Individual and the Organization*. Routledge.

Boud, D., Keogh, R. and Walker, D. R. (1985). *Reflection: Turning Experience into Learning*. London: Kogan Page.

Burtonshaw-Gunn, S. A. (2008). *The Essential Management Toolbox*. Chichester, West Sussex: John Wiley and Sons.

Carnell, C. (2007). *Managing Change in Organisations*. 5th ed. Harlow, England: Financial Times Prentice Hall.

Cole, G. A. and Kelly, P. (2020). *Management, Theory and Practice*. 9th ed. United Kingdom: Cengage Learning EMEA.

Drucker, P. (1968). *The Practice of Management*. London: Pan.

Evans, C., Pearce, R., Greaves, S. and Blake, H. (2020). Advanced clinical practitioners in primary care in the UK: a qualitative study of workforce transformation. *International Journal of Environmental Research and Public Health*, 17(12), p.4500.

Gibbs, G. (1988). *Learning by Doing: A Guide to Teaching and Learning Methods*. Oxford Polytechnic: Further Education Unit.

Handy, C. (1999). *Understanding Organisations*. 4th ed. London: Penguin Books.

Hunt, J. W. (1992). *Managing People at Work*. 3rd ed. London: The McGraw-Hill Companies.

Huston, C. J. (2022). *Leadership Roles and Management Functions in Nursing: Theory and Application*. Lippincott Williams & Wilkins.

Iles, V. (2006). *Really Managing Health Care*. 2nd ed. Berkshire: Open University Press.

Jones, B., Horton, T. and Home, J. (2022). Strengthening NHS management and leadership. *The Health Foundation*. Available at: www.health.org.uk/reports-and-analysis/briefings/strengthening-nhs-management-and-leadership (Accessed 13 August 2025).

Jones, R. and Jenkins, F. (2006) *Managing and Leading in the Allied Health Professions*. Oxford: Radcliffe Publishing.

LaGanga, L. R. (2019). *Management Skills for Clinicians, Volume I: Transitioning to Administration*. New York: Business Expert Press.

Langer, J. (2022). Bureaucracy and the imaginal realm: Max Weber, rationality and the substantive basis of public administration. *Perspectives on Public Management and Governance*, 5(2), pp.122–134.

MacGregor, D. (1960). *The Human Side of Enterprise* (Vol. 21, No. 166, 1960). New York: McGraw-Hill.

Marquis, B. L. and Huston, C. J. (2009). *Leadership Roles and Management Functions in Nursing. Theory and Application*. 6th ed. Philadelphia: Wolters Kluwer/Lippincott Williams and Wilkins.

Marriner Tomey, A. (2000) *Guide to Nursing Management and Leadership*. 7th ed. St. Louis, Missouri: Mosby.

McCambridge, J., Witton, J. and Elbourne, D. R. (2014). Systematic review of the Hawthorne effect: new concepts are needed to study research participation effects. *Journal of Clinical Epidemiology*, 67(3), pp.267–277.

Merriam Webster Dictionary (2025). *Management*. Available at: MANAGEMENT Definition & Meaning - Merriam-Webster (Accessed 13 August 2025).

Mertens, S., Schollaert, E. and Anseel, F. (2021). How much feedback do employees need? A field study of absolute feedback frequency reports and performance. *International Journal of Selection and Assessment*, 29(3-4), pp.326–335.

Mintzberg, H. (1973) *The Nature of Managerial Work*. New York: Harper and Row.

Mintzberg, H., Quinn, J. B. and Voyer, J. (Eds). (1995). *The Strategy Process*. Harlow: Prentice Hall.

NHS (2025). *Fit for the Future: 10 Year Health Plan for England*. Available at: www.england.nhs.uk/long-term-plan/ (Accessed 13 August 2025).

Prottas, D. J. and Nummelin, M. R. (2018). Theory X/Y in the health care setting: Employee perceptions, attitudes, and behaviors. *The Health Care Manager*, 37(2), pp.109–117.

Saif, G. B. D. (2024). Toward a dynamic model of human needs. A critical analysis of Maslow's hierarchy. *International Journal of Multidisciplinary Approach Research and Science*, 2(3), pp.1018–1046.

Salsberg, E. and Quigley, L. (2017) *Achieving sustainable and appropriately trained health and social care workers for ageing populations. Health Employment and Economic Growth: An Evidence Base*. Geneva: World Health Organisation.

Schon, D. A. (1987). *Educating the Reflective Practitioner*. San Francisco: Jossey-Bass Foundation.

Seden, J. and Reynolds, J. (2003) *Managing Care in Practice*. London: Routledge.

Srinu, G. (2023). *Administrative Thought*. Shhalaj Publishing House.

Sully, P. and Dallas, J. (2005). *Essential Communication Skills for Nurses*. Edinburgh: Elsevier Mosby.

Weber, M. (1947). *The Theory of Social and Economic Organisation*. Translated by A. M. Henderson and Talcott Parsons. New York: Oxford University Press.

Whetten, D. A. and Cameron K. S. (2024). *Developing Management Skills, Global Edition*. 10th ed. Pearson Education.

Yukl, G. A. and Gardener, W. L (2020). *Leadership in Organisations*. 9th ed. Global Edition. Pearson.

CHAPTER 6

The effective manager

Management skills for the advanced practitioner

Carol L. Cox

Introduction

Effective management skills are essential within the practice arena of advanced practice. It is not just an issue of acquiring the knowledge for utilising the skills but also of putting them into practice; Wood and Varacallo, 2025, 2023). This is particularly essential not only when managing your own time but that of the individuals you delegate responsibilities to in practice. How you manage yourself and others makes the critical difference in patient care outcomes and patient satisfaction (Moy et al, 2023). The purpose of this chapter is to assist you in developing specific and personal management skills through a series of practical activities, some of which are reflective and others for implementation during practice. These may not be the skills that you might be expecting to develop as a manager, such as how to effectively manage a budget, or how to carry out an appraisal or a performance review interview. Instead, the focus of this chapter is on developing management skills in a more subtle but profound way: developing your own self-awareness so that you can manage yourself and others effectively. You may be wondering how that will help you to become a better manager but by the end of this chapter you will agree that the most important person to get to know well is yourself. This chapter functions as a guide to assist you in obtaining the knowledge, skills, and strategies that will give you realistic and mature confidence to be an effective manager. Keep in mind that effective advanced practice practitioners managing themselves and others combine strong leadership with high emotional intelligence, excellent communication, and strategic thinking to improve patient outcomes and support staff (JAAPA, 2025; Moy et al, 2023). They demonstrate integrity, adapt quickly to industry changes, and foster collaboration through delegation and mentorship. Key traits include technical expertise, conflict resolution skills, and a patient-centred, resilient approach.

Learning outcomes

At the conclusion of this chapter, you will be able to:

DOI: 10.4324/9781003609049-9

- Understand the concept of emotional intelligence and identify ways in which emotional intelligence principles can be applied to your own management practice.
- Reflect on your communication and management skills.
- Develop an insight into your own management skills through reflective practice.
- Identify your own strengths and areas for development.
- Learn how to identify situations which trigger emotional responses in you and develop strategies to manage these.
- Gain an insight into how your actions impact others.
- Understand the importance of adapting the way you manage according to individual situations.

This chapter will begin with some additional management theory, which supports the management theory chapter. The purpose of including the additional theory is to demonstrate the theoretical basis underpinning the activities and case studies that follow. The chapter will conclude with some key messages for you as a developing advanced-level practice manager.

Background

The key characteristics of an effective manager in healthcare, categorised by skill set and derived from the American Nurses' Association (2026), Charter College (2026), and Nebraska Methodist College (2025), are:

(1) **Leadership and Emotional Intelligence**
- Empowerment and Delegation: Effective leaders move away from micromanagement, instead empowering team members to operate independently and innovating to improve care.
- Building Trust: Acting with integrity and creating a supportive environment helps maintain high team morale.
- Emotional Intelligence: Recognising and managing their own emotions while empathising with staff and patients is crucial for building rapport.
- Mentorship: They foster professional growth by acting as a mentor, educating and guiding staff towards excellence (American Nurses' Association, 2026).

(2) **Communication and Collaboration**
- Clear Communication: They adapt their communication style to various groups, ensuring expectations are understood.
- Active Listening: Good listening skills allow them to understand staff concerns and improve patient care.
- Conflict Resolution: They act as mediators, resolving disagreements between staff and navigating complex team dynamics (Charter College, 2026).

(3) **Strategic and Operational Skills**
- Strategic Thinking: They balance direct care needs with long-term organisational planning and financial goals.
- Adaptability: They embrace changes in technology, policies, and procedures to keep teams on track.

- Analytical Skills: They are data-literate and use a logical, detail-oriented approach for decision-making (Nebraska Methodist College, 2025).

(4) **Personal Attributes**
- Resilience and Composure: They remain calm and composed in high-pressure situations.
- Integrity: They maintain high ethical, moral, and professional standards.
- Positive Attitude: A positive outlook helps maintain high team morale, even in stressful, fast-paced environments (Charter College, 2026).

(5) **Focus on Quality**
- Patient-Centred: They prioritise patient care and safety above all else.
- Continuous Quality Improvement: They look for ways to improve services, often by challenging the status quo and encouraging innovation (American Nurses' Association, 2026).

Salter (2024) indicated in 2024 that while managers have had a role within the National Health Service (NHS) since its inception, it is only within the last 30 years or so that clinicians themselves have become managers, leading and managing their peers. It has been 40 plus years now and it is seen that advanced practice practitioners have expanded their leadership skills and management expertise exponentially. Historically, looking back, The Griffiths Report (Department of Health and Social Security, 1983) led directly to the situation of clinicians, trained in their specialist clinical area, taking on the additional duties and responsibilities of managing teams and even entire departments. A delicate balance had to be achieved by clinical managers. Now, even more than before, they must balance the politics of the organisation with its targets and specific demographics as well as current governmental demands. In addition, they must maintain clinical and managerial credibility amongst their peers and continue to enable the consumer-oriented health service (Oland et al, 2020; Iles and Sutherland, 2002). Furthermore, they must ration increasingly scarce resources and ensure clinical and political accountability (Oland, 2020; Department of Health, 1998, 2000). This is quite a set of expectations for any manager.

How does an advanced-level practice clinical manager successfully negotiate the endlessly changing political landscape and ensure a cohesive, financially prudent service whilst maintaining a close working relationship with the people they manage? What set of specific skills is required to do all this? There are practical skills, often relating to resources, that can be learned on courses, such as how to write a business case, how to manage a budget, or how to shortlist and interview. What are far more difficult to learn, far more intangible, are the 'soft' management skills; skills such as managing people, knowing how to deal with conflict, or managing change effectively.

How does a manager even begin to develop these skills? The best way to start is by thinking about yourself: getting to understand yourself and how you relate to others.

Emotional intelligence – Emotional Quotient (EI – EQ)

There are numerous definitions of emotional intelligence (EI) including Emotional Quotient (EQ) which is similar to a person's Intelligence Quotient (IQ). EI and EQ primarily focus on the importance of one's own feelings and emotions and how these affect not only your actions but the feelings and actions of those around you (Ross, 2025; Marquis and Huston, 2009; Stuart, 2004).

> Emotional intelligence (EI) is the ability to recognize and regulate your emotions, read others accurately, and build healthy relationships. It relates to how much someone is willing to learn and grow. In 2024, EQ emerged as the #1 leadership skill for any executive, especially in a world where employee well-being and human-centered culture have taken center stage.
>
> (Ross, 2025: 1)

Stuart (2004) addresses emotional literacy and indicates that leaders with EI can identify feelings and emotions in themselves and others and manage and reason with their emotions. This sounds exceptionally challenging and there are ongoing debates in the literature as to whether EI is something that can be learned or whether it is an innate ability that some people possess and others do not. Salovey and Mayer (1990), recognised as the 'pioneers' of EI, suggested that EI is a skill that develops with age, that some people have a natural aptitude for and is therefore difficult to learn. They refined their theory down to four specific mental abilities, or emotional building blocks of EI:

(1) the ability to actively perceive and express your own emotions.
(2) the ability to integrate feelings and emotions into thought processes on demand, thereby facilitating an understanding of yourself and others.
(3) the ability to understand emotions and what they mean for you and others.
(4) the ability to regulate or manage your emotions (Vitello-Cicciu, 2003; Weisinger, 1998).

Conversely, Goleman (1998) argued that EI can be learned, although he agrees that it improves with age. He suggests that every person has a rational, thinking mind and an emotional, feeling mind, both of which influence how individuals act. Goleman (1998) identified five key elements of EI, like those of Salovey and Mayer (1990). These are reinforced today by other experts in the field of EI/EQ (Channell, 2025). Matthew Channell (2025) has articulated Daniel Goleman's EI theory as having five components:

(1) Self-awareness: being able to recognise and understand your emotions, moods, and drivers, as well as how these impact others.
(2) Self-regulation: the ability to control any disruptive emotions or responses.
(3) Motivation: a drive to work towards a common goal.
(4) Empathy: being able to understand and accept other people's emotions, moods, and drivers.
(5) Social skills: the ability to build relationships and networks through finding common ground (Channell, 2025; Goleman, 1998).

Applying Goleman's theories of EI to nursing, Reeves (2005) suggests that it is the self-regulation element of EI that allows nurses, regardless of their internal emotions, to work in a calm and professional manner during difficult or chaotic clinical situations. However, Goldman's theories of EI could equally be applied to Allied Health Professionals. Furthermore, it is important to note that managers with EI achieve objectives through their self-awareness which promotes productive, motivated, and equal workplaces (Channell, 2025).

Weisinger (1998) agrees that EI can be learned, developed, and directly applied to work situations. He suggests a six-step approach to developing your own EI:

(1) **Developing high self-awareness**: observing yourself in action and reflecting on what you see can help you to change and shape your actions appropriately.
(2) **Managing your emotions**: rather than suppressing your feelings and emotions, allowing yourself to feel and learning to understand and then manage your emotions can free you up to productively deal with difficult situations.
(3) **Motivating yourself**: having clarity about a task as well as drawing on external sources of support can help you to turn potential setbacks into positive outcomes.
(4) **Developing effective communication skills**: the wrong words or unclear messages can be damaging and so developing good, clear communication and listening skills is critical.
(5) **Developing interpersonal expertise**: being able to understand and analyse the many individual relationships you as a manager must build and maintain is key. You are then able to communicate at the right levels at the right time with the right people.
(6) **Helping others to help themselves**: a successful team comprises more than one person and so helping others to manage their emotions, communicate effectively, and become motivated is critical. Keeping your own emotional perspective and being a supportive listener can help others solve their problems and achieve their goals (Weisinger, 1998).

The aforementioned are reinforced by authors such as Ross (2025) and Channell (2025). Most of the activities in the next section of this chapter are designed to help you to develop some of these key elements of EI.

Activities to enhance learning

This section contains some activities which will help you to think and reflect; not just on your skills and abilities as a manager but also about factors that impact on how you might behave in certain situations. The activities will give you some insight into the decisions you make, why you make them, and how you might think about your management practice in a different way; perhaps even changing what you do.

Activity 1 Reflective self-assessment

For you to realise your full potential as a manager, it is essential for you to have a clear idea of your strengths and areas for development as well as having a reasonable idea of how others see you. This self assessment activity will not give you all the answers, but it will help. It will take a little time for you to complete this activity; however, your patience and honesty will pay dividends and give you significant insights.

Have three short conversations, one with each of the following:

(1) your manager.
(2) someone outside your organisation, like a peer or a mentor.
(3) yourself.

These are the sorts of questions you should ask yourself as well as your manager and peer:

What are my strengths as a manager?
Am I making the most of them now?
Which strengths might be more valuable to me in the future?
Which management skills or abilities do I need to develop?
Is the lack of these skills holding me back now? If so, why?
Is it possible that not having these skills might hold me back in the future?
How much do I really want to do something about them?
What achievements am I most proud of this year?
What things have motivated and enthused me this year as a manager?
What experience have I gained this year?
What have I learned from these positive experiences?
What things have frustrated me this year? (These might be things like conflict, changes taking a long time to implement, or things going badly.)
How did I respond to these at the time?
What have I learned from these experiences?
What are the things I would really like to achieve as a manager in the short and long term?

Make a note of the answers; do they differ in any way? Do you see any patterns? What do the responses tell you about yourself as a manager? Do you think you are less capable than your manager thinks you are? Or are you more confident about your abilities than others around you think you are? What do you think you need to do to change the things you do least well?

Activity 2 What do I think is important as a manager?

It can be helpful to identify what sort of manager you are by being clear about what you are ***actually*** focusing on in your work as a manager, rather than what you feel you ***should*** be achieving. It is natural for most managers to aim to facilitate their teams to achieve their overall objectives in a way which is efficient and effective, adhering to externally set targets, within budget, and in the meantime keeping your team happy and cohesive. However, this may not necessarily be what you are actually doing; these are inevitably competing interests and the nexus of all of these is where all managers wish to be but rarely are.

Figure 6.1 (Venn, 1880) shows a Venn diagram of competing interests, showing each interest equally balanced with all the others, both in terms of size as well as overlapping with each other. Achieving this is rare; in reality, most people move from focusing on different elements at different times depending on the situation as well as how they feel.

Draw your own competing interests' diagram by thinking about the four areas listed below; try to be honest about what is most important to you most of the time. There are no right or wrong answers, just honest ones. Try to do this activity by thinking about what you actually feel and do, rather than what you feel you ***should*** be doing (i.e., having an equal set of circles!).

Determine the size of each circle by how important you feel that aspect of your work is *to you*. You can do this by thinking about how much time and emotional energy you use in trying to achieve these outcomes. What makes you angry? What makes you happy? What makes you satisfied at the end of the day? Listening to your feelings can help you decide the size of each circle. Then decide which of the other areas that circle should overlap with and by how much. You may have additional competing interests that are not shown here which compete for your time and attention. Ensure you add these as this is *your* diagram!

(1) Reaching all targets: how important is ensuring that you meet all targets from within your own organisation as well as all government targets to you as a manager? How much time do you spend on making sure this happens and how much of the team's resources do you allocate to this? What prices are paid by you as an individual as well as by the team in the efforts to meet targets (Short, 2005; Reeves, 2005)?

(2) Maximising income and keeping within budgets: if you can increase income, how important is this to you and how much do you and your team focus on this element of the work? Do you like to keep within budget? Do you feel you will be harshly judged if you do not? Do you lose focus on other things in your attempts to maximise income and balance budgets?

(3) Achieve all operational requirements: do you focus on getting the job done, even if you do not always stay within budget and occasionally miss some targets? Is your focus the care of the patient and if it means going over budget a little, you feel able to justify this as you have done your job as a clinical team? What impact do you think this has on the team or the organisation as a whole?

(4) Keeping the team happy and cohesive: do you go out of your way to enable a close, effective, and smooth-running team, who work well together? You may ensure you get things done in this way, but you may sometimes go over budget a little, e.g., by getting holiday cover for the team, or you may miss some targets, even though you feel these are important. Do you focus on the team because you want to be liked (Marquis and Huston, 2009), or because you feel a close team is an efficient one?

Be honest with yourself when doing this activity. It will help you to see what is actually important to you and will help you to identify areas to reflect on.

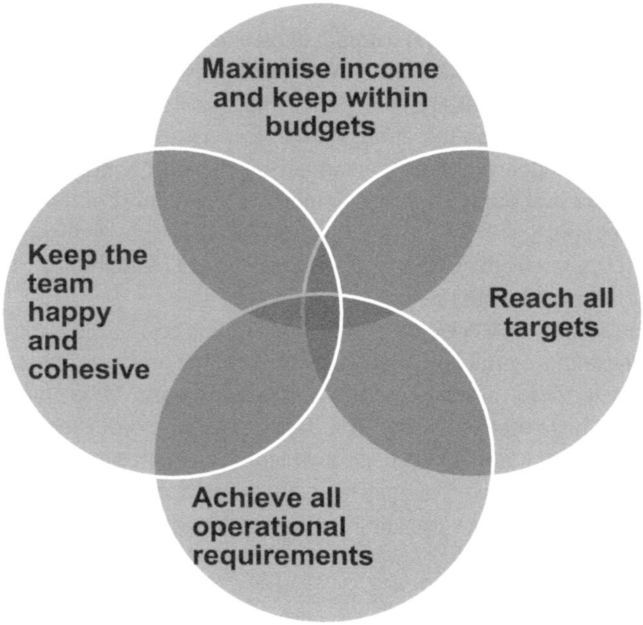
Maximise income and keep within budgets
Keep the team happy and cohesive
Reach all targets
Achieve all operational requirements

Figure 6.1 Example of a Venn diagram of balanced competing interests (Venn, 1880)

Using a learning journal

We all have preferred ways of doing things in the workplace and as a manager; we may not realise it, but we tend to do or respond to particular things in the same way most of the time. Some people or situations just press our buttons for one reason or another. Our reactions are entirely subconscious and instinctive. To develop as a manager one of the most powerful things we can do is to not only become *aware* of our 'buttons,' which are our preferred ways of doing things, but to gradually develop *choices* about how we do things or respond to situations (Short, 2005; BYU, 2025).

This is actually harder than it sounds; it means thinking critically and reflectively about things we have done or ways we have responded; particularly as it relates to relationship-building (Short, 2005; Browne and Keeley, 2006). We may not always like what we see but this ability to reflect on situations helps us to get to know ourselves better and to spot the patterns and drivers to our responses. The aim is to see and understand your patterns *the moment they occur* and then have choices about an appropriate response. Moving through these stages takes deep and honest reflection. A learning journal is a helpful tool you can use (Moon, 1999).

Try to keep your mind 'open' to significant events, interactions, or triggers during your working day. Some of these might include times when you have had a strong feeling or response such as excitement, boredom, frustration, feeling frightened, or feeling ignored. At some point in the day when something like this has occurred, make a little time to note the details briefly in a notebook. Come back to it later in the day or when you have a bit more time to complete the entry. You may simply be reflecting on your competing interests Venn diagram and finding that you have shifted your focus for some reason.

You may find that asking yourself the following questions helps you to focus on *you*: your role, responses, and actions in any given situation. The questions can also be used to help you to structure your journal entries.

What was going on? Play the event back in your mind; try to remember what exactly happened, who said and did what, any key phrases said by you or others, what the body language of all the players was. This is not about recalling the outcome but rather the details of the entire event.

How was I feeling at the time? Try to recall what you were feeling while the event unfolded: were you feeling anxious, excited, stressed, happy, or angry? Again, this is not always easy to do as we all have feelings we do not understand or acknowledge in ourselves. Being as honest as you can, when thinking about your feelings in a particular situation, will help you to see whether you respond in particular ways to certain feelings. Being aware of these automatic responses is the first step in changing those patterns.

What do I think this might mean? Can I make any connections here? Does this give me insights into how I respond in particular situations or what my triggers are?

What can I try next time? How can I actively make the choice to respond in a different way when something like this happens again? Are there any strategies I could use which would make me act more consciously (i.e., counting to ten before speaking or responding to a situation or waiting until the next day before responding to an email)?

Some tips on successful journal-keeping

(1) Try to make a detailed reflective entry in your journal around once a week if you can: it is not a diary so do not try to write something every day. Think of it as a process for you to use when there may be something for you to learn.
(2) Make the time to write your journal somewhere quiet when you will not be disturbed.
(3) Try to keep all your journal entries in one notebook, which is only used for that purpose.
(4) Once a month, go back and read through all the entries for that month in one go. Do you notice any patterns, any connections, and any particular triggers? If you do, what does this tell you about yourself? What have you learned about yourself? How might you do things differently next time? (Cannata, 2025; Healy and Murphy, 2023; Moon, 1999).

If you do manage to keep a regular learning journal and reflect on it on a monthly basis, you will find that you will be more aware of your feelings and responses and will start to 'be in the moment' much more. You will start responding in the way you would like to respond. You will also be much more aware of your own 'hooks' and 'traps': the people and situations which 'press your buttons' and to which you respond in a way that is emotional and raw rather than considered and of your choice.

Using reflective practice in meetings

We all have to attend meetings at times; some of us more than others. As a manager you may be responsible for chairing meetings and setting agendas. However, how many good and successful meetings can you truthfully say you have participated in? These were meetings in which everyone had their say; all matters on the agenda were appropriately dealt with in a timely fashion and clear decisions were made?

Certainly, one of the most satisfying moments at work is when you experience being part of a group working well together to solve a problem. Conversely, being part of a team which does not quite gel or does not get on top of a problem can be one of the most frustrating experiences at work. It is not uncommon to feel anxious about being excluded, blamed, or insecure about our position in a meeting which is not well chaired. If you feel like this then it is likely that others may feel something similar, despite the Chair's best efforts to include everybody and cover the agenda comprehensively.

Think about effective meetings that you attend. What does the Chair do to make them effective? Looking at the following lists before and after a meeting (particularly if you are chairing) will help you to reflect more on your role in meetings and how you prepare for them and give you the tools to be an effective chair.
Things to think about *before* a meeting

(1) What is the purpose of the meeting?
(2) Are the right people invited? How well do they know each other?
(3) Does the agenda reflect the purpose of the meeting? Can anything be taken off? Does anything need to be added?
(4) Are there to be full minutes or just action points?
(5) Does any information need to be distributed in advance? If you want people to discuss and reach an agreement about, say, a lengthy policy, they need to see it ahead of the meeting.
(6) Who will lead each item on the agenda? It is a good idea to delegate agenda items to those best able to give the relevant information or lead the discussion. Agree in advance who will lead which discussion.
(7) Do the agenda items 'flow' well? It can be helpful to start with something easy and quick, with more difficult and long items in the middle and ending with shorter, 'clarifying things' items.
(8) Do not spend ages reviewing previous minutes, be familiar with the minutes and the agenda, and be clear and concise about what is being carried forward onto the current agenda.
(9) How do you move between agenda items? Summarise the discussion and remind people of the decision.
(10) How do you keep to time? If a discussion has gone on longer than planned, consider suggesting coming back to the item next time, giving people a task to prepare for a decision at the next meeting. An example would be asking everyone to check what the preferences are within their team or asking someone to get more information for next time.
(11) Be aware of shifts of energy as well as body language. Are people tired or bored? Can you bring that discussion to a prompt conclusion and move on to another agenda item?
(12) Be aware of your own feelings; others may be feeling the same.
(13) How do you end the meeting well? Quickly review the actions, decisions, and next steps and thank people.

(14) Always finish on time!

Asking yourself the following questions *after* the meeting can also be helpful in giving you insight into the dynamics at the meeting as well as how you dealt with it.

(1) Who spoke most? Who spoke least? Why?
(2) Was the time spent on each agenda item used well? If not, how could that item have been dealt with more efficiently?
(3) Did people listen to each other and discuss matters openly?
(4) Which actions or people helped the meeting flow well?
(5) What actions or people do you think hindered the meeting's progress the most?

(Browne and Keeley, 2006)

Your responses to these questions and subsequent reflections will be telling and interesting. Consider trying something different at the next meeting: experiment with ideas and structures or test your hypotheses by carefully looking to see if the same response occurs in a similar situation.

Reflecting on your power

There are many types of power that you, as an advanced-level practice manager, have and use (ANA, 2023; Farrington, 2007). There are, however, numerous factors which may contribute to how much power you think you have as well as how much power other people *perceive* you to have. Some of these factors may seem obvious or trivial at first glance; some of them you will have control over while others are an innate part of you, or even a product of society's assumptions or expectations. Regardless, they are important for you to think about when trying to work out how others see you or experience your authority. Activity 3 can help you think about your power as a manager.

Activity 3 Look at the following list and think about what effect, if any, the factors below have on your power as a manager.

(1) **Gender**: are you 'given' more power because of your gender and if so, why? Do you 'take' more power because of your gender? Why? How does this interact with the gender of the people being managed?
(2) **Nationality:** do you share the same nationality with some members of the team? What impact does that have on your power?
(3) **Educational background:** does having a similar social or educational background with some members of the team give you a special bond?
(4) **Looks:** Does attractiveness give someone more or less power? Does wearing a suit (for men or women) mean that someone is given or takes more power?
(5) **Height:** can someone short have as much 'presence' as someone tall? If so, why?

(6) **History within the organisation:** how important is it to have been working in the organisation for longer than others in the team? Or for significantly less time?
(7) **Experience:** does having more experience in your specialist area give you more power? Is it you who takes that power or others that give it to you?

(Adapted from Morgan, 1989; O'Regan and Ghobadian, 2004.)

Understanding your power activity

Think about your current management role and functions, on a daily basis, and complete this over a period of one month. Come back to sections even when you think you have finished and will not make further changes or additions. Use this space to jot down your thoughts and any examples.

	How much of this power do I have?	*How often do I use this power?*
	None, some, a lot	Never, sometimes, often
Positional or Legitimate Power Do you have formal authority in your role? (i.e., take decisions or supervise other people)?		
Connection Power Are you close to someone who is powerful within the organisation and other people know you know them? Do you know powerful people outside the organisation?		
Resources Power Do you have control over resources: pay, promotion, training budgets, annual leave?		
Expert Power Do you have specialist knowledge or qualifications?		

(Adapted from Morgan, 1989.)

Case studies

Case studies are accepted as an innovative and thoughtful learning resource for managers in all fields of practice (ANA, 2023; Vitello-Cicciu, 2003; Mayo and Thompson,

1995; Salovey and Mayer, 1990). It is well documented that people can learn more effectively when actively involved in the learning process (Sivan et al, 2001; Bonwell and Eison, 1991). The case study approach is one way in which such active learning strategies can be implemented.

There are a number of definitions for the term case study. For example, Fry et al (1999) describe case studies as complex examples which give an insight into the context of a problem as well as illustrating the main point. In this chapter, a case study is defined as a person-centred activity based on topics that demonstrate theoretical concepts in an applied setting.

The following section has been compiled to help you to reflect on some of the more theoretical elements of this chapter as well as how you tackled and completed the practical activities. You will be able to apply some of the things you may have learned about yourself and about organisations to some practical scenarios.

Some of these scenarios position the participants in contexts which may be familiar to you; even if you do not recall a similar incident, it is likely that you will have faced similar personal or professional dilemmas. By working through the case studies, you can reflect on what *you* would have done if you had been in that situation. This will help you to apply your knowledge of EI/EQ to resolve practical problems and issues and make thoughtful and appropriate decisions.

Case study 1

Josie is a newly appointed advanced practice clinical nurse manager in a long-established palliative care nursing team with a sound reputation in an inner-city borough. Josie is new to the area and applied for the job as a sideways move, having already managed a similar but slightly smaller team in a different area. Part of the attraction of the job was how highly regarded the service is, as well as getting an opportunity to work with other experts in her chosen clinical field. The person who had previously held the management job had been in post for over five years and was an experienced manager and palliative care practitioner.

Josie's new team welcomed her warmly and were helpful and supportive in her first week. However, Josie felt anxious that she was somehow perceived as less experienced than her predecessor and in her first team meeting felt insecure and shy when talking about her vision for the service. Her team were unclear about the changes that Josie was proposing and responded negatively, expressing their concerns about changing things that they perceived to be working well. As the meeting progressed, Josie felt more defensive and less certain about her proposals and suggested that the team come back to the discussion after she had been able to get more information.

Josie wrote about the meeting in her learning journal and reflected on what had happened and how her feelings of inadequacy had led to her shyness and lack of confidence in the meeting. She reflected on whether she was indeed less experienced than her predecessor and was clear that she was as experienced, if not more so. For the next meeting, Josie prepared thoroughly, gathering data to support her proposals for change and approached the subject clearly and confidently. She used statements such as 'I think this is a good idea because...' and 'I think that our new rota will give patients an excellent service because....' The use of a personal statement such as 'I think.' helped Josie to clarify what she was thinking as well as recognising and reiterating that she is the person responsible for the service. By not saying that the new rota would provide *better* patient care, Josie reassured the team that she was not critical of the existing levels of patient care. This reduced their negativity towards her. Her preparation and confidence in presenting her vision for the service further inspired her team to get behind the proposed changes.

Case study 2

Paul shares a caseload with his colleague, Sam, but they work in different offices on the same floor and often use the same files, just at different times. Paul feels that he is careful to ensure that he always returns the files after he has used them but finds that Sam hangs onto files on his desk, meaning that Paul spends time looking for them in the drawer and then must go and look on Sam's desk or ask for them when he needs them. Despite Paul's regular requests to Sam to put the files back in the drawer once he has finished them, Sam continues to hold onto files regularly. Paul feels angry, disrespected, and that Sam never listens to him. Every time he looks for a file and cannot find it he feels angry. It is affecting how he responds to Sam at other times.

Sam does not understand why Paul is so grumpy in the office all the time and assumes that Paul does not like him. He also begins to wonder if Paul's grumpiness is because he is getting burnt out clinically but decides to keep an eye on things and not discuss his concerns with a manager yet.

Paul attends a course where he is encouraged to keep a reflective journal. After a month of entries, Paul reads his journal and notes that he has been writing as much on his anger towards Sam as on the care of the patients on his caseload. Paul decides he must take some action and starts to pay close attention to how he responds each time he finds that Sam has not returned a file to the drawer. He realises that once he has one negative thought about Sam such as 'why doesn't he listen to me?', a 'domino effect' of feelings follows. He finds himself thinking further negative thoughts towards Sam such as 'what is wrong with him?', 'he is so selfish,' or 'I wish he would just leave.'

Paul realised that he was generalising about Sam and making wild interpretations of Sam's behaviour. He thought carefully and realised that Sam is actually not selfish in other ways, and he certainly listens to Paul and respects his opinion when they discuss patients or other matters. He decides to tell Sam how upsetting he finds not being able to find files when he needs them. Paul talks about how hard he finds the situation, and how frustrating and time-consuming it is and asks Sam if there is some way they can resolve the matter. Paul even suggests that he would be happy to come and get the files from Sam's office once he has finished them if he lets Paul know when he is done with them.

Sam is astonished that Paul feels so strongly about the files and is immensely relieved that a simple solution can be found to his absent-mindedness. Understanding how upsetting Paul finds not being able to find shared files makes Sam more conscious of what he does with files when he has finished with them and over a short period of time, their working relationship improves hugely.

Conclusion

In this chapter you have learned how important it is to have a sound awareness of your own feelings and how these can impact on your behaviour, as well as that of others.

Keeping a learning journal for reflection can be a valuable tool and doing this regularly over a minimum of one year can help to identify any patterns in your feelings or behaviour in particular situations. Although there is no magic formula for becoming the perfect manager, these final points serve as reminders and may be helpful:

(1) Step back and notice what is happening around you: reflect on the dynamics of every interaction you are part of before speaking or acting.
(2) There is no need to have a personality transplant: know your strengths and weaknesses, reflect on these, and work to change your responses.
(3) Get help with reflection: get a mentor, join a peer support group, and keep a reflective diary.
(4) If something is not working, try a new strategy.
(5) Your management style may need to differ and adapt according to the person or situation.
(6) Being a good listener makes you a better advanced-level practice manager.

Acknowledgements
The editor would like to thank Raf Benato for her contribution to the first edition of the book, we have built on her works in this new edition.

References

American Nurses' Association (2026) General Insights in Nurse Leader Competence and Retention, 1 CEU www.nursingworld.org/continuing-education/MP2025P616/ (Accessed 2/11/2026).

ANA Nursing Resources HUB (2023) How to Be a Good Nurse Manager. September 15, 2023. www.nursingworld.org/content-hub/resources/nursing-leadership/a-good-nurse-manager/ (Accessed 2/8/2026).

Bonwell, C. C. and Eison, J. A. (1991) *Active Learning: Creating Excitement in the Classroom*. ASHE-ERIC Higher Education Report No. 1. Washington, DC: The George Washington University, School of Education and Human Development.

Browne, M. and Keeley, S. M. (Eds.) (2006) *Asking the Right Questions: A Guide to Critical Thinking* (8th edition). New Jersey: Prentice Hall.

BYU (2025) Engaging with Messy, Emotional, Personal Side of Writing: Can Learning Journals Enhance a Student's Writing Experience? Brigham Young University, 19 (2025). https://locutorium.byu.edu/issues/volume-19-2025/engaging-with-the-messy-emotional-personal-side-of-writing-can-learning-journals-enhance-a-students-writing-experience/ (Accessed 05/06/26)

Cannata, S. (2025) 10 Journal Prompts for 2026 and How to Start a Journal. www.sarahcannata.com/10-journal-prompts-for-2026-and-how-to-start-a-journal/ (Accessed 2/8/2026).

Channell, M. (2025) Daniel Goleman's Emotional Intelligence. TSW Training, October 6, 2005. www.tsw.co.uk/blog/leadership-and-management/daniel-goleman-emotional-intelligence/ (Accessed 2/10/2005).

Charter College (2026) What Traits Do the Best Healthcare Managers Have? https://chartercollege.edu/news-hub/what-traits-do-best-healthcare-managers-have/#:~:text=Your%20positive%20attitude%20is%20one,improve%20patient%20care%20and%20outcomes (Accessed 2/5/2026).

Department of Health and Social Security (1983) *The NHS Management Enquiry. Griffiths Report*. London: HMSO.

Department of Health (1998) *A First Class Service: Quality in the New NHS*. London: HMSO.

Department of Health (2000) *The NHS Plan*. London: HMSO.

Farrington, J. (2007) *Top 7 Sources of Personal Power*. Available at: http://Top7Business.com/?expert=Jonathan-Farrington (Accessed 30/08/2010).

Fry, H., Ketteridge, S. and Marshall, S. (1999) *A Handbook for Teaching and Learning in Higher Education*. Glasgow: Kogan Page.

Goleman, D. (1998) *Working with Emotional Intelligence*. New York: Bantam Books.

Healy, N. and Murphy, C. (2023) Case Reports, Reflective Practice and Learning to Succeed. *Anaesthesia Reports*, 11(1):e12212. doi: 10.1002/anr3.12212

Iles, V. and Sutherland, K. (2002) *Organisational Change: A Review for Healthcare Managers, Professionals And Researchers*. London: NIHR Service Delivery and Organisation Programme. Available at: www.healthknowledge.org.uk/sites/default/files/documents/publichealthtextbook/5c/5c2_review.pdf (Accessed 05/06/26).

JAAPA (2025) A Blueprint for NP and PA Leadership. *Journal of the American Academy of Physician's Assistants*. Sullivan Cotter, October 31, 2025. https://sullivancotter.com/jaapa-blueprint-np-and-pa-leadership/#:~:text=Health%20systems%20science%20(HSS)%20is,Leading%20Others (Accessed 2/11/2026).

Marquis, B. L. and Huston, C. J. (2009) *Leadership Roles and Management functions in Nursing: Theory and Application* (6th edition). London: Wolters Kluwer Health/Lippincott Williams and Wilkins.

Mayo, M. and Thompson, J. (1995) *Adult Learning: Critical Intelligence and Social Change*. London: National Institute of Adult Continuing Education.

Moon, J. (1999) *Learning Journals: A Handbook for Academics, Students and Professional Development*. London: Kogan Page.

Morgan, G. (1989) *Images of Organisations*. London: Sage.

Moy, H. P, Giardino, A. P. and Varacallo, M. A. (2023) Accountable Care Organization. StatPearls Publishing; Treasure Island (FL): July 25, 2023. (Accessed 2/6/2026).

Nebraska Methodist College (2025) 10 Traits of Effective Healthcare Leadership, January 10, 2025. www.google.com/search?q=Nebraska+Methodist+College+(2025)+10+Traits+of+Effective+Healthcare+Leadership&rlz=1C1CHBF_enUS747US765&oq=Nebraska+Methodist+College+(2025)+10+Traits+of+Effective+Healthcare+Leadership&gs_lcrp=EgZjaHJvbWUyBggAEEUYOdIBCDIwNjZqMGo0qAIAsAIA&sourceid=chrome&ie=UTF-8&zx=1770585451626&no_sw_cr=1 (Accessed 2/9/2026).

Oland, E. et al. (2020) A Framework of Nurses' Responsibilities for Quality Healthcare – Exploration of Content Validity. *Science Direct*, Elsevier, 27(2): 150–163.

O'Regan, N. and Ghobadian, A. (2004) Leadership and Strategy: Making It Happen. *Journal of General Management*, 29(3): 76–92.

Reeves, A. (2005) Emotional Intelligence. *American Association of Occupational Health Nurses Journal*, 53(4): 172–176.

Ross, M. (2025) Developing Your Emotional Intelligence for That Executive Role in 2026. *Leadership Forbeswomen*, December 9, 2025. www.forbes.com/sites/mariaross/2025/12/09/developing-your-emotional-intelligence-for-that-executive-role-in-2026/ (Accessed 2/8/2026).

Salovey, P. and Mayer, J. D. (1990) Emotional Intelligence. *Imagination, Cognition and Personality*, 9(1990): 185–211.

Salter, B. (2024) *The New Politics of Medicine*. Basingstoke: Palgrave Macmillan.

Short, L. (2005) Why Emotional Intelligence Is Critical for Successfully Managing Up. Harvard University, Professional and Executive Development, Harvard Division of Continuing Education. August 28, 2025. https://professional.dce.harvard.edu/blog/why-emotional-intelligence-is-critical-for-successfully-managing-up/#Why-Do-Middle-Managers-Need-Emotional-Intelligence (Accessed 2/8/2006).

Sivan, A., Wong, L. R., Woon, C. and Kember, D. (2001) An Implementation of Active Learning and Its Effect on the Quality of Student Learning. *Innovations in Education and Training International*, 37(4): 381–389.

Stuart, P. (2004) Emotional Intelligence: Developing Emotionally Literate Training in Mental Health. *Mental Health Practice*, 8(4): 12–15.

Venn, J. (1880) On the Diagrammatic and Mechanical Representation of Propositions and Reasonings. *Philosophical Magazine and Journal of Science*, 9(59): 1–18.
Vitello-Cicciu, J. M. (2003) Exploring Emotional Intelligence. *Journal of Nursing Administration*, 33(4): 203–210.
Weisinger, H. (1998) *Emotional Intelligence at Work*. San Francisco: Jossey Bass.
Wood, M. L. and Varacallo, M. A. (2023) Management Skills, NIH National Library of Medicine, StatPearls Publishing, LLC (Accessed 2/6/2026).
Wood, M. L. and Varacallo, M. A. (2025) Management Skills, 2nd edition, NIH National Library of Medicine, StatPearls Publishing, LLC (Accessed 2/6/2026).

CHAPTER 7

Advanced nursing practice in the United States of America

Managing, negotiating and monitoring the healthcare system

Jane Sumner

Introduction

This chapter will enable you to critically discuss and explore the role of the advanced practice nurse (APN) in healthcare delivery in the United States of America (USA), the different specialties of advanced practice nursing, and the various organisations that influence/control it. Advanced nursing education is included, as is practice with all the issues the nurse must consider and attend to as he/she negotiates a fraught professional landscape. To negotiate the system, nurses need to be cognisant of major issues that relate to licensure, accreditation, certification and education (LACE) for advanced practice because they influence where nurses will practise and how they will practise. Barriers to practice that relate to advanced nursing practice satisfaction are also discussed.

Learning outcomes

At the conclusion of this chapter, you will be able to:

- Understand the changes in education for APNs and the expectation of competency in evidence-based practice.
- Explicate population health and the social determinants of health.
- Examine the implications of COVID 19 on nursing education and nursing practice.
- Articulate the multiple pressures influencing advanced practice nursing in the USA.
- Differentiate the different licensing, accreditation, certification, and educational issues associated with APN practice in the USA.
- Comprehend issues related to negotiating and managing practice as an APN.

Background

In the USA the population is ageing and unlike the United Kingdom (UK), in which healthcare is provided free via the National Health Service (NHS), fewer Americans have

DOI: 10.4324/9781003609049-10

healthcare insurance coverage which limits access to service. Chronic disease management is becoming more problematic with increasing obesity and its attendant illnesses, e.g., diabetes mellitus, hypertension, and cardiovascular disease. However, Healthcare Reform became federal law as the *Patient Health Protection and Affordable Care Law* and the *Health Care and Education Reconciliation Practice Act* in March 2010. This changed to a degree how healthcare is delivered (Public Health Law 111–148, 2011). This law forces a paradigmatic shift from episodic, acute illness care to health promotion, wellness, disease prevention, and optimal management of chronic disease. It has opened opportunities for APNs as never before – providing they are willing to take advantage of the change. The ongoing shift is inexorably towards primary care in neighbourhood clinics, and a 'medical home' for every American citizen. APNs who have specialised in geriatrics, family, adult, paediatrics, and women's health are well positioned for practice in the delivery model.

There is a realisation that all nurses and particularly APNs must have an education that addresses the social determinants of health (SDOH). Millet (2022) cites *Healthy People 2030* which provides a strategic framework for a national agenda. It explicates core epidemiology principles that communicate methodologies for improving health and achieving health equity. The overarching goals include improving wellbeing by preventing disease, eliminating health disparities, achieving health equity, and enabling an individual to achieve his or her full potential. Focusing on acute health care, which is downstream care, does not enable the nurse to ensure that his or her patients can achieve these goals.

The Future of Nursing 2020-2030 (2021) makes very clear that there has been too much emphasis in education on acute nursing care which is practised in hospitals with little in the curricula that focuses on population health and health equity. Acute health care is downstream care and population health is upstream healthcare which means there must be a focus on the SDOH. Nurses have different opportunities with upstream healthcare with home healthcare, school nursing, public health nursing, work in prisons, rehabilitation agencies, hospice, and many other community sites as well as the emergence of telehealth. There must a shift back into the community or at least care outside the acute care hospital.

Atkins and Szanton (2025) when discussing the redesign of nursing education refer to Florence Nightingale who lived in the mid-to-late 19th century as someone who understood the importance of a clean environment, clean air and water, and healthy diet. Lillian Wald, one of the founders of the Henry Street Settlement, coined the phrase 'public health nurse,' and of whom there is a famous photograph of her clambering between the roofs of tenements in New York City in the late 19th century. She is wearing a long dress and a hat and carrying a black bag. This latter continues to be carried by visiting nurses. She is practising 'community as clinic.' Both women can thus be said to understand the social determinants of health and how these effect individual patients and communities. They were both public health nurses.

Atkins and Szanton (2025) affirm that the 'community as a clinic' is where advanced practice nursing education should be housed. Atkins and Szanton (2025) further indicate this optimises nurses' contribution to healthier, and more equitable resilient communities. In order to do this, the following must be done:

(1) Expand the areas in which nurses consistently work
(2) Diversify the demographic makeup of the nursing workforce to mirror the nation's diversity
(3) Ensure nursing graduates are well prepared in a variety of settings

Within the arena of measurable competency-based education, there are both 'psychomotor and higher-order conceptual skills' or 'critical thinking' skills. In addition, it involves being aware of 'cultural sensitivities,' communication abilities with the healthcare team and the patients and families.

Population health is far more than a segment of the populations with a particular health problem, e.g., children's health. The aim must be improving health equity and the social determinants of health as the influencers on overall population health. The USA is a culturally diverse country, with many different values, beliefs, and biases. It is also an ageing population. Chronic diseases are problematic in all ages and in all races, i.e., black, Hispanic, Caucasian, or Asian. These are issues that must be addressed in nursing education.

The SDOH include: income, on which so much of life depends; food insecurity, too many people live in a 'food desert'; housing instability, which can mean not being able to pay the rent, and/or descending into homelessness; transport needs, where the population is dependent on public transport; utility needs, which can mean lack of heat in the winter, or lead in old water pipes, such as what occurred in Flint, Michigan in 2014. Utility needs also include regular trash pickup. Neighbourhoods may not be safe for children to be outside playing. *Culture of Health,* 2014 was published by the Robert Wood Johnson Foundation with a focus on enabling the US population to lead 'healthier lives' by removing obstacles that affect 'the health and the well-being of individuals' (Millet, 2022). This means directly addressing SDOH.

A rural population can have different needs from an urban one. Just access to the internet and WiFi can be problematic for this population. Access to healthcare: whether it is a physician, an APN, a clinic, or a hospital is another problem for some rural populations. Physical health is not the only issue for APNs to address, but also mental health and dental health. Government policies influence factors in good health, e.g., The Affordable Care Act (2010) enabled many who prior to the passing of this act had no access to healthcare because of lack of income or having a job that did include health insurance. Changes in Medicaid coming in late 2026–2027 will affect a considerable number of Americans who have no other access to healthcare.

The shift to primary care raises concerns because of the ongoing and projected shortage of primary care doctors. In 2008, only 2% of all new doctors selected primary care as their specialty (Hauer et al., 2008). Unfortunately, by 2030, 20% of the American population will be more than 65 years old (He et al., 2005) and historically it is the older population that has greater need of healthcare services. APNs are increasingly 'filling this gap while maintaining quality care and often lowering health care costs' (Stanley et al., 2009) and presumably continue to do so. One study by Brooten et al. (2023) studied five groups of patient problems and the difference APNs made in terms of improving patient outcomes. The most important function of the APN was surveillance of physiological and psychosocial needs, and the patient's environment; followed by health teaching; guidance and counselling; case management; and finally treatments and procedures. These functions reduced hospital length of stay and home visits assisted in preventing readmissions for considerable cost savings. What this suggests is that the APN is providing quality primary healthcare with excellent patient outcomes, cost-effectively. As Stanley et al. (2009) state:

> Nurses are arguably in the best position to realize the goals of health care reform, which include enhancing access to affordable care, providing patient-centred care, focusing on wellness and prevention, improving quality and outcomes of care, emphasizing chronic illness management, assisting patients in making informed choices, and improving care coordination.
>
> (Stanley et al., 2009)

Advanced practice nursing

APNs in the USA are registered nurses (RNs) who have received masters-level (graduate) education, which is built on baccalaureate education and practice. There are many specialties to select from, and like in the UK, APNs may practise independently or in an interprofessional team, in acute care or non-acute care. Within acute care, APNs may practise in specialised units, e.g., in different intensive care units, the emergency room, or specialty outpatient clinics (i.e., pain management or diabetes management). In the non-acute environment APNs may practise in long-term care, specialty rehabilitation facilities, community health/neighbourhood health clinics, public health/community health, schools, prisons, retail-based clinics, or occupational health.

Many RNs in the USA, as in the UK, select the graduate education that builds on their practice experience (i.e., the nurse who works in a neonatal intensive care unit may well decide to become a neonatal nurse practitioner). Others will opt for something quite different, i.e., the nurse who has run a large outpatient clinic may choose to become a public health/community health nurse. In the USA, those nurses who decide they want to become a Certified Registered Nurse Anaesthetist (CRNA) are required to have practised in a surgical intensive care unit for a designated period before being admitted to that specialty educational programme and are certificated in Advanced Cardiac Life Support (ACLS).

The APN is an independent, autonomous practitioner, practising under his/her own licence. The acronyms APN and APRN (i.e., Advanced Practice Registered Nurse) are equally accepted by the State Boards of Nursing (Easom, 2005) as descriptors of nurses who have received nursing education and have acquired certification and/or licensure as an APN (APRN, 2008). There are, however, many different types of, or titles for APNs to further confuse the issue: Clinical Nurse Specialist (CNS); Clinical Nurse Leader (CNL), this nurse is regarded as a generalist practising at an advanced level and who remains in acute hospital practice; Advanced Practice Registered Nurse (APRN); Nurse Practitioner (NP); Certified Registered Nurse Anaesthetist (CRNA); Certified Nurse Midwife (CNM); and more recently the Doctor of Nursing Practice (DNP). Within the 'nurse practitioner' nomenclature, there are further subspecialties, i.e., Family Nurse Practitioner (FNP) or Geriatric Nurse Practitioner (GNP). In addition, the APN may become certified in any one of a number of specialties that do not have required specialist licensure, i.e., enterostomal nursing or oncology or palliative care nursing.

Some of these specialties will be eligible for prescriptive authority, e.g., NP, or, not e.g., CNS. Each of the 50 states and the District of Columbia allow for some form of prescriptive authority. In some states APNs have limited prescriptive authority, usually within some sort of organisational protocols, like the Patient Group Directions (PGDs) used in many NHS Trusts in the UK. Other states permit unfettered prescriptive authority, and still other states will allow unfettered prescriptive authority except for the ordering of narcotics. Prescriptive authority covers not only the ordering of medications, but also the ordering of laboratory tests and durable medical equipment. Some APNs will indeed practise truly autonomously and independently, but others will practise under a doctor or in collaboration with one. Some APNs will practise in acute hospital care and others will practise in non-acute care sites. The expectation of the APN regardless of title and education is to: be a leader of the interprofessional team; enable nurse colleagues to utilise evidence-based practice principles; communicate effectively with all members of the team including patient and family (Tuite and George, 2010). Studies reveal that most patients in the USA are satisfied with the care they received from APNs, and in some instances more than satisfied with APN care than that received from doctors or physician assistants (Agosta, 2009). This is mainly because of their holistic approach to both patient and family and particularly in shared medical appointments (Watts, et al., 2009). This finding is a similar finding in the UK (Cox et al., 2010; Cox and Hall, 2007).

Activity 1

Consider Chapter 1, From the Beginning to Advanced Practice, An Expanded Historical Narrative, in this book. Issues were raised regarding the variety of titles associated with the APN role. Issues were also raised regarding regulation (licensure) of practice. What issues do you see in relation to the aforementioned? Are there lessons that can be learned from the USA?

Licensure, accreditation, certification and education (LACE)

Understanding advanced nursing practice in the USA has become increasingly complex, partly because of the different organisations weighing in on different aspects of it: whether it is legislative or regulatory, this latter includes 'educators, certifiers, and licensing bodies' (Stanley et al., 2009:341). These organisations include the American Association of Colleges of Nursing (AACN) (AACN, 2011) and the National League for Nursing (NLN), which accredit schools of nursing; specialist certification bodies, e.g., American Nurses Credentialing Center (ANCC); the licensure organisation the National Council of State Boards of Nursing (NCSBN, 2021) with individual state boards; the National Association of Clinical Nurse Specialists (NACNS) which has identified core competencies required of all CNSs and is developing core education requirements; and finally, different specialty organisations. A number of recent reports from the Institute of Medicine (IOM) (To Err is Human, Institute of Medicine, 1999; Crossing the Quality Chasm, Institute of Medicine, 2001; Priority Areas for National Action: Transforming Healthcare Quality, Institute of Medicing, 2003a; Future of the Public's Health in the

21st Century, Institute of Medicine, 2003b; Who will Keep the Public Healthy, Institute of Medicine, 2003c) make clear that the USA cannot continue with its highly dysfunctional healthcare delivery system, which is fragmentary at best, very expensive, and has some of the worst health indices of the developed world. These reports reveal concerns about access to healthcare services, the quality of services, the quality of organisations which have their own scope and standards of practice, e.g., the National Organisation of Nurse Practitioner Faculties (NONPF), or the American Academy of Nurse Practitioners (AANP), or the Council of Anaesthesia (COA).

Although evidence-based practice has been the underpinning of all levels of nursing education for some years now, the AACN (2021) published its revised *Essentials: Core Competencies for Professional Nursing Education* to include competencies in skills and knowledge in evidenced-based practice, which are measurable, and which are demonstrated before graduation. All graduation programmes must include at least 500 hours of clinical experience in which the student must demonstrate competence. Population health and the SDOH are now a focus, and the student must demonstrate competence in this as well.

As stated previously, there are reports from the Institute of Medicine (IOM which reveal concerns about access to healthcare services, the quality of the services provided, and what needs to be done to improve them. Five core competencies have been recommended to be included in the education of all healthcare professionals (HCPs) and to be implemented in practice. These are (Finkelman and Kenner, 2007):

Provide patient-centred care
Work in interdisciplinary teams
Employ evidence-based practice
Apply quality improvement
Utilise informatics

Partly, but not only because of these reports, 44 national nursing organisations came together to reach a consensus on what APRN regulation should be. A working group was formed that produced the Consensus Document, which is supported by the NCSBN(2021) and has become the standard for LACE. There were four goals established by the working group which are (Stanley et al., 2009:344):

To strive for harmony and common understanding in the APRN community to promote quality APRN education and practice
To develop an agreed-to vision for APRN regulation, including education, accreditation, certification, and licensure
To establish a set of standards that protect the public, improve mobility, and improve access to safe, quality APRN care
To produce a written framework that reflects consensus on APRN regulatory issues and strengthens the APRN position within the healthcare system

Within the Consensus Document, the APN roles have been identified as Nurse Anaesthesia, Nurse Midwife, Clinical Nurse Specialist, and Nurse Practitioner. The population foci are: family/individual across the lifespan, adult gerontology, neonatal, paediatrics, women's health/gender related, and psychiatric mental health. Other specialisations, i.e., oncology or palliative care, or orthopaedics, are also included in APRN practice, provided the nurse has received graduate education in the specialty. What is not specifically included in the Consensus Document is that nursing administration and public health/community health nursing are not regarded as APRN practice specialties. However, as Stanley et al. (2009) attest, the Consensus Document has not yet been fully implemented, and its success ultimately is contingent on national acceptance and implementation. This seems to suggest that there may still be room for negotiation, but that is by no means clear. The concerns for those in nursing administration and public health nursing rest on the issue of advanced courses in health assessment, pathophysiology, and pharmacy (3Ps) that are necessary knowledge for APRNs, but which are not curricula content or necessary for practice in these two specialties.

Not only does AACN accredit schools of nursing within its arm the Crediting Commission Nursing Education (CCNE), but so does the National League of Nursing within its National League for Nursing Accrediting Commission (NLNAC). It seems however that the AACN Essentials document has had a greater influence on graduate nursing education than the NLNAC and therefore it is the model utilised most frequently. From an educational perspective the AACN has mandated the Essentials of Master's Nursing Education, which provides the required curricula content and also the framework of a school's organisational structure. Meeting the Essentials is required of schools accredited by CCNE (refer to Table 7.1).

The Consensus Document has already been adopted by the NACNS, as it developed core educational competencies required for CNSs. These educational competencies have been derived from the Three Spheres of Influence in Patient Care: the Patient/Client Sphere; the Nurses/Nursing Sphere; and the System/Organisational Sphere (Goudreau et al., 2007:311) that constitute practice competencies domains. They stated that 'clinical expertise in a specialty is the hallmark of CNS practice … [having] clinical expertise

Table 7.1 Essentials of Master's Nursing Education

Essential	*Scientific Underpinnings for Practice*
Essential I	Background for Practice from Sciences and Humanities
Essential II	Organisational and Systems Leadership
Essential III	Quality Improvement and Safety
Essential IV	Translational Scholarship for Evidence-Based Practice and Innovation
Essential V	Information Systems/Technology and Patient Care for the Improvement of Health Care
Essential VI	Health Policy and Advocacy
Essential VII	Interprofessional Collaboration for Improving Patient and Population Health Outcomes
Essential VIII	Clinical Prevention and Population Health for Improving Health
Essential IX	Master's-Level Nursing Practice (Advancing Professionalism and Professional Values)

Source: (AACN, 2011) American Association of Colleges of Nursing Master's Essentials

in diagnosis and treatment used to prevent, remediate or alleviate illness and promote health within a defined specialty population' (Goudreau et al., 2007:311).

In 2021 AACN published its new *Essentials* with a shift from Evidence-Based Practice to Competency-Based Practice. Both Masters and Doctoral (DNP)-level nursing education must address SDOH, social justice, disparities, and health equity. For the first time AACN acknowledges the APN specialities that are nursing administration leadership, informatics, public health/population health, and health policy. The new *Essentials* include ten Domains and seven Concepts for nursing education for both undergraduate and graduation levels:

Domains		**Concepts**
Domain 1.	Knowledge for Nursing Practice	Clinical Judgement
Domain 2.	Person-Centred Care	Communication
Domain 3.	Population Health	Compassionate Care
Domain 4.	Scholarship for Nursing Practice	Diversity, Equity & Inclusion
Domain 5.	Quality and Safety	Ethics
Domain 6.	Interprofessional Partnerships	Evidence-Based Practice
Domain 7.	Systems-Based Practice	Health Policy
Domain 8.	Informatics and Healthcare Technologies	Social Determinants of Health
Domain 9.	Professionalism	
Domain 10.	Personal, Professional, and Leadership Development	

In addition, *2021 Essentials* state that there are two levels for practice; level two is for advanced practice nursing 'sub-competencies' which are specific to the different specialities, i.e., CNM or CRNAs. These revised *Essentials* have the state boards of health in mind as these license all nurses.

State boards of nursing

The power of the state boards of nursing (BON) should never be underestimated because of their policing responsibility to keep the public safe. Each of the BONs in the 50 states and the District of Columbia have regulatory control, which means these organisations have final responsibility for controlling practice authority, reimbursement, and prescriptive authority. Each BON has its own Practice Act, which has been passed by its State Legislature and is periodically reopened for necessary and timely changes. Each BON is made up of nurses from different aspects of the profession, e.g., practice and education. The governor of a state makes the final selection of BON members and in many states a term lasts for four years. The BON meets monthly to discuss issues of concern that relate to policing and regulation. This body has the responsibility of licensing nurses but also of removing nurse's licences for egregious actions (like the Nursing and Midwifery Council [NMC] in the UK). In the case of (suspected) egregious actions, the nurse is given a fair hearing to ensure that all the evidence is considered before a punishment (if required) is decided. Thus, the ultimate autonomy of the APN rests with the BONs that decide the professional's ability to be able to make decisions within the limits of the education, skill, and professional competency of the provider which results in efficient use of resources (4).

In 2021 the National State Boards of Nursing (NSBN) published its revised Model Act which states the act 'shall be known and may be cited as the Jurisdiction Nurse Practice Act (NPA) which creates and empowers the board of nursing (BON) to regulate nursing and to enforce the provisions of the Act.' The APN is clearly defined as a person who has had basic nursing education, as well as graduate-level APN education at a school that is accredited by a national accrediting board, and has certification from a certifying body. In addition, the APN must have 'one population focus.' The six population foci are: family/individual across the lifespan; adult-gerontology; neonatal; paediatrics; women's health/gender-related; or psychiatric/mental health. The NSBN clearly define the APN's scope of practice, including prescribing medications.

In 1973, Idaho became the first state to pass legislation granting APNs 'supervisory, collaborative, and independent authority to practice' (Phillips, 2010:24). Since then, every state has followed suit although the degree of responsibility and autonomy varies from state to state. There is no federal right of control over state rights in this instance. It is the state that grants licensure and prescriptive authority to the individual Advanced Nurse Practitioner (ANP). This means that as an ANP moves from state to state he or she must be cognisant of the rules and regulations for practice of the state in which he or she is practising.

In recognition of a need for an APN to cross state lines to practise in an emergency or to practise telehealth across state lines, several states worked together to establish in 2020 what is now known as the 'Advanced Practice Registered Nurse Compact,' which enables the APN to be registered in one state and practise in another state within the Compact. The APN is required to fulfil all the obligations of the regulating state of licensure. To clarify, a licence can be renewed in the 'home' state and the APN can automatically have reciprocity in another Compact state. Presently, additional states are joining the Compact.

Scope and standards of practice

The scope and standards of practice of many different specialties, at both general and specialist levels, have been published by the American Nurses Association (ANA) as well as many specialty organisations. These essentially define the competencies expected of all APNs, as well as the limits of a specialty practice (ANA, 2007). The role of ANPs is defined by the Scope and Standards of Nurse Practitioners (AANP, 2002) as 'they … are primary care providers … Nurse practitioners practice autonomously and in collaboration with health care professionals and other individuals to diagnose, treat and manage the patient's health problems' (American Academy of Nurse Practitioners 2002b cited by Weilland, 2008). Refer to Table 7.2 (AACN, 2011) for the Domains and competencies for Nurse Practitioners (NPs) that have been produced by the National Organisation of Nurse Practitioner Faculties (NONPF, 2006; 2022). These Domains and competencies correspond with the Domains and competencies produced by the NMC (2005) and the Royal College of Nursing (RCN, 2011).

Table 7.2 Domains and Core Competencies of NPs

Domains	*Core Competencies*
One	Management of Patient Health/Illness Status
Two	The Nurse–Practitioner–Patient Relationship
Three	The Teaching–Coaching Function
Four	A Professional Role
Five	Managing and Negotiating Health Care Delivery Systems
Six	Monitoring and Ensuring the Quality of Health Care Practice
Seven	Culturally Sensitive Care

Source: (NONPF (2022) National Organisation of Nurse Practitioner Faculties Domains and Core Competencies of Nurse Practitioner Practice (2006).

According to Stewart et al. (2010), the AANP in its 2007 *Standards of Practice* document outlined 'qualifications, process of care, care priorities, collaborative responsibilities, documentation requirements, patient advocacy responsibilities, quality assurance, adjunct roles, and research initiatives' (Stewart et al., 2010:27) for all NPs. The emphasis is on NP responsibility, comprehensive assessment, and decision making.

Individual nurse practice within a specialty can be evaluated according to the specific standards regardless of which organisation provides them (i.e., COA, NONPF, or ANA). The ANA's Public Health Nursing Scope and Standards of Practice are provided in Table 7.3 (ANA, 2007) as an example of specific specialty standards.

Master's preparation or Doctor of Nursing Practice

Unfortunately, the nurse who is seeking advanced practice has many issues to confront when selecting an education programme which will drive future practice. No longer are the choices limited to a master's degree, largely because of the number of clinical practicum hours required of NP and CRNA education; thus, increasing the total number of credit hours required for graduation. The AACN proposed that a DNP degree should be the degree of choice, particularly for the two specialties mentioned. The AACN is calling for all schools that offer these two specialties to provide a DNP by 2015. However, AACN is not limiting this degree to only CRNAs and NPs. Rather it indicates that there are two different patient care foci for this degree: direct patient care which requires all these APNs to have completed the 3Ps, and indirect patient care which does not require the 3Ps; so, all specialties are included. This means that both nursing administration and public health/community health nursing will also be included in DNP degrees.

There have been several arguments posited on why the nursing profession needs to have a DNP. One of the leading reasons has been to achieve parity with other healthcare professions, i.e., pharmacy, physical therapy, occupational therapy, and audiology. Another reason is how advanced education improves patient outcomes. The number of credit hours required in certain specialties to achieve this, e.g., CRNA, is more than required for a regular master's degree. Furthermore, the salary has the potential to be higher. Upvall and Ptachcinski (2007) compared nursing with pharmacy. They discovered that nursing initially led the way towards this advanced degree, but it was pharmacy who in fact introduced a professional doctorate before nursing. The primary rationales for a PharmD degree were a 'societal healthcare need that occurred as pharmacotherapy

Table 7.3 ANA's Public Health Nursing Scope and Standards of Practice

Public Health Nursing Competencies	*Scope and Standards of Public Health Nursing Practice*	*Standards of Practice for Public Health Nursing*
Proficiency: Advanced Mastery of the competency. Individuals are able to synthesise, critique, or teach the skill Domain 1 Analytic Assessment Skills Domain 2 Policy Development/ Programme Planning Skills Domain 3 Communication Skills Domain 4 Cultural Competency Skills Domain 5 Community Dimensions of Practice Skills Domain 6 Basic Public Health Sciences Skills Domain 7 Financial Planning and Management Skills Domain 8 Leadership and Systems Thinking Skills	Tenets 1 Population-based assessment, policy development, and assurance processes are systematic and comprehensive 2 All processes must include partnering with representatives of the people 3 Primary prevention is given priority 4 Intervention strategies are selected to create healthy environmental, social, and economic conditions in which people can thrive 5 Public health nursing practice includes an obligation to actively reach out to all who might benefit from an intervention 6 The dominant concern and obligation is for the greater good of all of the people or population as a whole 7 Stewardship and allocation of available resources support the maximum population health benefit gain 8 The health of the people is most effectively promoted and protected through collaboration with members of other professions and organisations	Standard 1: Assessment Standard 2: Population Diagnosis and Priorities Standard 3: Outcomes Identification Standard 4: Planning Standard 5: Implementation Standard 5A: Coordination of Services Standard 5B: Heath Education and Health Promotion Standard 5C: Consultation Standard 5D: Regulatory Activities Standard 6: Evaluation Standards of Professional Performance Standard 7: Quality of Care Standard 8: Education Standard 9: Professional Practice Evaluation Standard 10: Collegiality and Professional Relationships Standard 11: Collaboration Standard 12: Ethics Standard 13: Research Standard 14: Resource Utilisation Standard 15: Leadership Standard 16: Advocacy

Source: ANA (2007).

became an increasingly important component' (Upvall and Ptachcinski, 2007:317) and the increasing knowledge of pharmacology, pharmacokinetics, and clinical pharmacotherapy. Similar rationales can be provided for nursing, and pharmacy has provided nursing with the necessary direction.

Although AACN has mandated the DNP in lieu of the traditional master's degree by 2015, there is debate on the wisdom of this and whether some specialties would be better served by only offering a master's degree or perhaps both degrees. Avery and Howe (2007) discuss the pros and cons of a Master's in Nurse-Midwifery versus a DNP because of a survey of 110 CNMs. The results revealed that although the Directors of Midwifery Education have endorsed AACN with a position statement (that has several caveats) there seems to be no resolution on the appropriate course of action, and there are insufficient data to date to support a DNP. Because a DNP would take longer than a traditional master's degree issues related to increased cost were raised, and whether as many nurses would apply for a DNP in Nurse-Midwifery, which would further increase the shortage of CNMs. More practicum hours would be required, and this could further stress what is already a difficulty in finding enough clinical sites and appropriately prepared preceptors. However, 68 of the surveyed nurses did indicate that they believed a DNP would increase their stature. Present DNP programmes already address AACN's Eight Essentials. Whether to move from a master's degree to a DNP further confounds the problem for this specialty because not all midwives are nurse-midwives. They are certified midwives who have not completed the nursing component in a school of nursing.

This chapter reveals some under-discussed issues as schools move from the traditional master's programmes, be they CNS or APRN, to the DNP. Length of education and cost are serious considerations, and upon graduation whether there will be jobs available with commensurate salaries. For associate degree prepared nurses (ADN) who aim for graduate education these problems are even greater as they must move through the different educational levels (Bachelor of Science Degree [BSc]; Master of Science [MSc]).

Activity 2

Reflect on your present level of education and training. Is it essential for you to obtain additional education and training to achieve your goal of becoming an ANP? If 'yes,' at what level should your education and training be directed?

Identify the current pros and cons to obtaining an ANP qualification. Are you able to take action now? If 'yes,' what initiatives are required for you to act?

If you are presently practising as an ANP, what level of education and training do you have? Is it sufficient to maintain your position as an ANP? If 'no' what additional education and training do you think is required?

Practice issues

The nurse, having made the decision on a specialty practice and an educational programme, has more issues to confront on graduation. He or she must consider where he/she wants to practise and whether prescriptive authority is something he/she believes he/she must have, and he/she must find the information to ensure the right decision is made.

Once educated and licensed as an APN, then where to practise becomes the central issue. Furthermore, the APN will have to confront barriers that confound that practice. This is more so in the very fluid healthcare delivery world, which is currently the USA system, as healthcare reform goes from enacted law into policy, rules, and regulations. If the new APN is going to practise within a collaborative doctor practice, then should that APN charge under his/her own licence and credentials, or should he/she bill under the collaborating doctor's name?

Regardless of the changes that are coming, at the present time the newly minted APN in the USA is required to take the specialty certification examination; apply for state licensure; consider how he/she will achieve the continuing education credits for re-licensure; take out malpractice insurance; ensure the number of annual practice hours that are required for ongoing certification; understand billing and reimbursement issues, along with the different reimbursement mechanisms depending on who the third-party payer is; and if planning to open an independent business then develop a business plan and ensure that it is not undercapitalised, if it is going to be sustained.

For those APNs who are going to practise within facilities that are accredited by Joint Commission (which accredits acute care facilities and many non-acute care facilities, i.e., home health agencies in the USA), then they will have to undertake the process of credentialling and privileging. Credentialling refers to the 'process of verifying education, licensure, and certification to practice as an advanced practice nurse, whereas privileging involves granting the authority to perform specific aspects of patient care' (Kleinpell et al., 2008:279). Scope of practice is underscored by the process of credentialling and privileging and ensures that the nurse meets the standards of the specialty of the position sought, and that the nurse is indeed educated, licensed, and certificated for that position; if not then the APN is unable to work in that position. Credentialling and privileging 'promote [s] accountability, enforce[s] professional standards of practice, enable[s] third party billing for services, and communicate[s] the scope of practice to other professionals' (Kleinpell et al., 2008:279). Increasingly the potential employer will require a criminal record check (CRB) of the candidate and can request the [federal] National Practitioner Data Bank provide information regarding 'licensure disciplinary actions, malpractice payments or adverse actions affecting professional memberships' (Kleinpell et al., 2008:280). According to Joint Commission accreditation requirement the APN must be evaluated regularly with reappointment two to three years post-hire if appropriate. The six competencies now required by Joint Commission in relation to medical staff, and which APNs must now meet are: 'patient care skills; medical knowledge, interpersonal and communication skills, professionalism, practice-based learning and systems-based practice' (Kleinpell et al., 2008:286).

For some APNs a Convenient Care Clinic (CCC) may be the practice site of choice in partnership with other APNs. These clinics are not uncommonly located in shopping malls, and treat minor acute illnesses 'such as sore throats, upper respiratory infections, fevers, rashes and urinary tract infections' (Evans, 2010:24), but no chronic illnesses, with flexible hours 24 hours a day 7 days a week. Evans stated that these clinics 'offer convenience, value, location, quality and cost' (Evans, 2010:24), and reduce pressures on overcrowded emergency rooms (accident and emergency departments) and urgent care clinics. All patients are charged small, cash-only rates which are posted outside the clinic, no credit cards accepted – which is important for those patients with no health insurance. Some APNs prefer rural practice rather than urban practice, and indeed they may be the only healthcare providers in many underserved rural states.

One small, convenience sample study completed in the northeastern USA demonstrates the practice of NPs in a variety of non-institutional settings. Deshefy-Longhi et al. (2008) present results from electronic data collection of the 54 NPs who chose to participate. These nurses were practising in paediatric, family, adult, women's health, and geriatric practice: most of which were home visits to the elderly in assisted living facilities; in private paediatric and obstetric clinics; and in community-based clinics. Most of the visits by patients were for acute health problems, with 'only 30% of visits for chronic illness management (either routine care or treatment of an exacerbation) and even fewer for health promotion' (Deshefy-Longhi et al., 2008:286), but the NPs did provide routine screenings and annual checkups. However, the NPs offered health promotion and disease prevention teaching and counselling; particularly in comparison with doctors who participated in similar electronic data collection studies. Interestingly, these nurses prescribed medication in 63% of cases for the acute problem visit and for the primary diagnosis. Anything more specific would depend on the NP's specialty and his/her patient population (i.e., the paediatric population would be different and have different needs from the geriatric population). 40% of reimbursement came from Medicaid, self-pay (because of no healthcare insurance), or no pay, suggesting the bulk of these nurses' patients were poor and/or minority patients. The limitation of this study is the small sample and the patient populations seen. However, it does provide an indication of a typical NP non-institutional practice (Deshefy-Longhi et al., 2008).

Third-party payers and reimbursement

Obviously, the APN expects to be paid for services rendered but how this is set up depends on the state, the type of practice, and the type of specialty. In the USA there are two 'public' sources of funding for healthcare services.

The federal government funds Medicare which is medical insurance available for those over the age of 65 years. It is complicated by the fact that different parts pay for different services: Part A pays for hospital services for when a person is an inpatient, and Part B pays for doctor services on an outpatient basis. The latter requires significant monthly co-pay. Part C is a combination of both Medicare Parts A and B generally offered at a lower cost to the original Medicare but is administered by private insurance companies who put the patient into a network with specific doctors and hospitals, which may limit services. Part D is the medication coverage component, but this has limits in coverage. Medicare only reimburses for 80% of the cost of services provided. This means that those who can afford it will have ongoing private insurance which will pay 80% of the outstanding 20% of the bill. Patients are required to pay some sort of co-pay, and this can be variable. Under the 1997 Federal Balanced Budget Act Medicare was authorised to reimburse APRNs (including NPs, CNSs, and CRNAs) at all practice sites, but at rates that were only 85% of doctor rates (Mercer Ray, 2008).

Medicaid, which largely provides care for the indigent, is a state-run healthcare-financing organisation that decides what service in a particular state will be covered (i.e., how much is reimbursed for home care, how much is reimbursed for days in an acute care hospital, how much to reimburse doctors, but is supported with both federal [the majority amount] and state funding). Many APNs are reimbursed under Medicaid, but if in solo practice may or may not be reimbursed under Medicare. In some Medicaid state programmes, the APN is reimbursed for services at 100% of the doctor fee, and in other states the APN is reimbursed at only 70% or 80% of doctor fees.

Medicaid is a programme of medical insurance specifically for children called the State Children's Health Insurance Programme (SCHIP) which is a combination of both federal and state monies. This means that all children without healthcare insurance have access to services including routine vaccinations and checkups.

One other federal programme that both provides services and pays for them is the Veterans Health Administration (VHA), which is available nationwide. Services covered include in-hospital care, rehabilitation, nursing home, home health, doctor and APN services, and some medication assistance. Veterans of wars with no other health insurance are eligible for services, and in some instances so are their families. Those who return wounded from ongoing wars are not initially included in the VHA, but once they are discharged from military hospital services, they are. Studies demonstrate that VHA patients are satisfied with APN services and job satisfaction amongst these nurses is high as well (Faris, et al., 2010; Watts et al., 2009). In fact, Watts et al. (2009) stated that the turnover rate of APNs in the VHA system was low at 7.8% for APNs and 5.7% for CNSs, which suggests APN satisfaction in practice compared to regular staff nurses working outside the VHA system who had a turnover rate of 8.8%. Faris et al. (2010) discussed that when practice was in a shared medical appointment environment, the overall patient outcomes when managing chronic illness were better than most other models. They stated that this model, when utilised in managing hypertension, diabetes, and heart failure, meant patients and families played a bigger role in their self-management and decision making. The APN was a change agent with good communication skills who worked well with the team.

There are many dozens of companies that provide health insurance to Americans (De Navas-Walt et al., 2010). In recent decades there has been an effort to rein in healthcare delivery costs and two new identities emerged that have tried to do so: health maintenance organisations (HMOs) and preferred provider organisations (PPOs) are examples of groups trying to control cost; essentially by not treating patients or by limiting what will be covered. Many employers who provide their employees with health insurance will decide which HMO they offer. A HMO will have its own doctors and hospitals under contract, usually at some sort of discounted rate, and all those enrolled in these organisations will have to select from the contracted providers. Some companies pay for APN services, others may not. The traditional health insurance companies are fee-for-service, but these are becoming less common, although they do cover all services provided.

What this means for the new APN is that he or she must be aware of the business end of service provided, and this may well drive whether practice is collaborative, in a group with doctors and other specialists, or whether the APN goes into practice with only other APNs. If the APN remains within a hospital system, it may or may not separately line-item his/her services. Regular registered nurse services are not a line-item in a hospital budget or on invoices submitted to the third-party payers. The APN must be knowledgeable about reimbursement issues in the particular specialty in which he/she is practising.

The irony is that despite the plethora of groups funding healthcare, there are still more than 46 million people without healthcare insurance in the USA, and who thus technically have no access to healthcare services unless they are willing to pay out of pocket. Few can afford this. It was this glaring need that the recent healthcare reform law was trying to address.

Activity 3

Identify the advantages and disadvantages of working as an independent ANP. Besides specific malpractice insurance coverage, what other expenses are incurred in independent practice?

Prescriptive authority

Prescriptive authority includes the ordering of medication, controlled or otherwise, the ordering of laboratory and other tests, and ordering durable medical equipment. By and large prescriptive authority, which is granted by individual states, is only given to those nurses who are NPs and who have completed the courses in the 3Ps. According to Mercer Ray (2008) CRNAs do not prescribe in the administration of giving anaesthesia, although this is not necessarily true if they are managing pain. Since 2000, nurse-midwives have had some prescriptive authority in all 50 states and the District of Columbia. The 50 states differ in how they will allow NPs to prescribe medications: 'In 47 states NPs can prescribe controlled substances, although some states limit the amount the quantities prescribed or place other restrictions on this prescribing' (Mercer Ray, 2008:555). Only five states give NPs unencumbered status in relation to controlled substances: Arizona, Montana, Oregon, Washington, and Wyoming as well as the District of Columbia. All APNs who have prescriptive authority must apply and be issued with a Federal Enforcement Agency (FEA) number, which is theirs alone and must be written on all prescriptions. In some instances, the CNS has limited prescriptive authority, and the NACNS supports this as a 'discretionary option' (Mercer Ray, 2008:555), but this is usually within narrow institutional protocols.

Activity 4

If you are a nurse prescriber, what (if any) are the limitations on your prescribing privileges? Do you see a need to change these privileges? If 'yes,' in what way should they be changed?

Barriers to practice

Unfortunately, there remain barriers that lead to the underutilisation and recognition of APNs. Many of these are politico/socio/economic. As Weilland (2008) stated, 'the factors of physician dominance, reimbursement, and state rules and regulations have created practice environments that are detrimental to full recognition of NPs as autonomous practitioners' (Weilland, 2008:345). This leads to '(a) denial of primary provider status, (b) decreased patient access to care, and (c) increased healthcare costs' (Weilland, 2008:345). What emerges from the nursing literature is that doctor dominance and resentment, and perhaps their failure to understand what APNs do, are one of the most serious threats to independent and fully autonomous APN practice. Some doctors have claimed that, compared to themselves, APNs have had too little graduate education to be able to practise independently and/or responsibly, that APNs aren't safe, do not refer appropriately and in a timely fashion, and finally, doctor supervision and collaborative practice are a must (Partin, 2009). Multiple studies in the nursing literature make clear that none of these reasons are completely valid, and in some instances the APN makes fewer errors than either the doctor or physician assistant (PA). This latter entity may be regarded as the true 'doctor extender' rather than the APN who is sometimes referred to as such. However, this has led some commentators to state that NPs have been seen as 'doctor extender' and 'cheap labour' because NPs improved physician productivity and income as each billing incident 'realized 100% reimbursement' (Weilland, 2008:347). This negates the APN as a primary care provider who emphasises health promotion and stresses the '"*medical*" role as a physician substitute' (Weilland, 2008:347). In many respects this is insulting, if not outright humiliating, to the autonomy of the APN. The American Academy of Family Practitioners (2006) has stated that APNs should be supervised by doctors, otherwise a 'second-class system of health care' will emerge (cited by Weilland, 2008:348). Weilland also claimed that the Committee of Pediatric Workforce has also opposed independent ANP practice, prescriptive authority, and reimbursement. What this suggests is that doctors retain enormous power, privilege, and prestige but are fearful of any loss of economic benefits. What is ironic about this, according to Phillips (2010), who did a meta-analysis of the literature, is that NPs demonstrate high-quality, safe patient care, and health outcomes and resource utilisation that are equivalent to doctors. At the same time patients remain highly satisfied with NP services.

The state BON, as the licensing authority, and the rules and regulations within the State Practice Acts are highly controlling of APN practice and particularly when it comes to prescriptive authority. Thus, BONs may be seen as barriers to APN practice. This should probably be interpreted cautiously because of the public's safety and the BON responsibility. However, Fontana's (2008) dialectical analysis of APN prescribing reveals that APNs are judiciously cautious when prescribing, and when it comes to narcotics may not or refuse to prescribe them at all. In some instances, because of fear of being prosecuted, they will ignore patients' need for narcotics to treat non-malignant chronic pain. This study suggests that innate APN caution is a barrier.

What does not seem to be discussed very often in the literature is that many healthcare facilities do not seem to understand exactly what the scope of practice is for both the APN and the DNP. Heinen et al. (2019) completed a review of leadership competencies and attributes in advanced nursing practice. Beeber et al. (2019) noted that these nurses are prepared for leadership roles, but this is not always utilised by the facility because the scope of practice is not fully understood or accepted. According to Li et al. (2023) the new APN may not be completely cognisant of his or her full scope of practice. It will take time to grow into the role.

Technology is and will continue to impact APN care, e.g., robotics and Artificial Intelligence (AI). What is not mentioned however is genetics and genomics. The question to be answered is medical research is largely functioning at the genetic level and cures or changes to various illnesses will no doubt impact APN practice. Will the role move into more of a counsellor and teacher role in the community? Spinal Muscular Atrophy once meant children not living into adulthood. Now with prebirth treatment these children will survive and develop almost normally. How will the APN support families with more than one child with SMA and the overall cost of treatment? AI in nursing practice is now emerging. Raymond et al. (2022) identified 11 articles that met their criteria and that AI aided NP clinical decision making and improved the effectiveness in data interpretation. These authors caution that in the articles they investigated all sites would be described as 'developmental' or 'experimental,' but not yet fully adopted. Vasquez et al. (2023) discuss in their review of the literature technology and AI and the implication for nursing practice, not only for advanced nursing practice. Different articles from different countries reveal that AI can improve nursing practice because it enables the care to be more patient-centred. But the caveat is that robotics can take over many of the tasks and skills performed at present by RNs. This causes fear in nurses about job safety in future. But these authors attempt to be reassuring by stating that nurses are innovative, creative, and imaginative. And finally, nursing is about humanness and making the human-to-human connection. AI is about the digital revolution and thus must be accepted as part of the next step forward in patient care.

COVID 19 in 2020 was the most recent pandemic in a century that had a devastating effect in the US and on the nursing profession. As is well known initially there was a national shortage of personal professional equipment (PPE), and this put nurses at great risk when caring for highly infectious patients. Initially there was no vaccine which would help protect nurses. The death rate amongst nurses was alarming. A study by Sonney and Peck (2023) on paediatric APNs demonstrated without doubt that it was not APNs who were affected by caring for those with COVID 19. There were 1087 nurses in this study and 87% reported professional burnout, 80% reported concern for their own health, and concern related to the mental health of children was 90%. In personal communication with intensive care nurses during the pandemic this author heard them state: 'everlasting fatigue;' 'death after death every day;' and anger at dying patients who hadn't bothered to get the vaccine once it was available. This latter did not affect how they practised professional nursing, they practised utilising their professional selves but found it hard to share much in the way of personal self. This was a protective mechanism; they were burned out but still went on working. But according to Ladak and Sasinski (2021) the pandemic enabled CNSs to expand their practice in hospitals with their crisis management skills during this public health disaster for which the country was inadequately prepared. They identified issues relating to supplies, workflow management, decision making to improve difficult situations, and leading hospital rounds. O'Reilly-Jacob et al. (2022) discuss how during the pandemic 22 states allowed a temporary full practice authority; the APNs had more control over their practice enabling telehealth practice, or more expedited care. However, these authors state that there is a need for regulatory frameworks that ensure the APN is fully practising within their scope of practice, particularly at times of emergency as with the COVID 19 pandemic. They stress that the current scopes of practice are outdated.

Schools of nursing had to change their teaching methods quickly. Students couldn't physically attend lectures: faculty were no longer able to be in the school in their offices, they had to work at home. Video lecturing and interactive assignments had to be quickly set up. Faculty as well as students had to learn new methods of ensuring the quality of education was not diminished (Kennedy-Malone et al., 2023). These efforts included clinical-based videos that focused on topics like managing a frail elderly patient, progressive fatigue, or end of life issues; all of which proved effective in learning. Some of the videos were posted on YouTube. Students were required to watch the video in its entirety and then tested. Results suggested that videos would be continued in the curriculum. Hospital clinicals were out of the question, nurses were overwhelmed with desperately ill patients, and the risk of infection was too high for students. Online simulation became the norm and proved to be effective. There was concern however that online clinical simulation was not the complete answer. Advanced practice nursing education required a significant number of clinical hours. Five hundred hours is the least number of clinical hours required by AACN and for specialties like registered nurse anaesthetist clinical hours are significantly more. McIltrot et al. (2022) discussed how one school included instruction in telehealth because in practice this was increasingly having to be utilised. Chike-Harris et al. (2022) ensured that students in telehealth also learned the relevance of being credentialled and licensed and how to bill for services. Another school that offered the CRNA programme learned the COA was concerned about how the students would learn all the necessary procedures needed. These included: mask management; tracheal intubation; alternative trachea intubation/endoscopic techniques; endoscopic techniques; spinal; epidural; peripheral nerve blocks; arterial puncture/catheter insertion; central venous insertion catheter placement; and intravenous catheter placement. Having gone through the official departments of 'US Department of Education, and the Council for Higher Education Accreditation, as well as statements related to COVID-19 and its impact on clinical education released by other nursing accrediting accreditors' (Bricker et al, 2022) it was accepted that simulated experiences could be up to '20% of 10 of the 17 required anaesthetic methods and skills' (Bricker et al, 2022).

If nothing else, what all nurses learned from COVID 19 was the importance of caring for self. This pandemic proved the critical role of nurses in maintaining all healthcare services and without them there isn't service. All nurses were the true heroes and hopefully are given more recognition for the vital contribution they made. APNs regardless of specialty demonstrated leadership day after day, supporting their colleagues. One study by Osborne et al. (2022) revealed that nurses working in cancer units during COVID 19 were fatigued and stressed, but a fellowship programme that was created to support these nurses who were transitioning to cancer units was effective and they developed more resilience and compassion as a result. According to Wood et al. (2022) moral distress during COVID 19 was higher with acute care practitioners but all nurses, whether in Upstream facilities or Downstream facilities, suffered some degree of moral distress. It seems safe to say that all nurses during the pandemic regardless of the site suffered but as stated were the heroes who went to work every day regardless of the personal toll. Lessons learned during COVID 19 have now been incorporated into master's and doctoral programmes for ANPs.

Conclusion

This chapter has demonstrated that if you are contemplating working as an ANP as a career choice, you must be a highly informed consumer if you are to negotiate and manage your advanced practice in the USA. This can also be said of advanced practice in the UK and perhaps other countries as well. Changes in policies, rules, and regulations are occurring so rapidly that remaining informed is imperative. Your career will hinge on what you select as a programme of graduate study, followed by licensure and certification requirements if you choose to practise in the USA. From there, decisions related to the type of practice you wish to pursue, whether it is within an acute care facility or in some type of non-acute care community-based organisation, whether to pursue solo practice or practise with another APN, or whether to join in a collaborative doctor practice must be examined. Reimbursement is a thorny issue, and unfortunately it has been relatively common for APNs to be practising with a poorer population, who may or may not have healthcare insurance. Third-party payers have not always reimbursed at the same rate as doctors. For NPs there is also the issue of prescriptive authority. They must be fully cognisant that this is granted by a state and is not transferable to another state. The newly mandated federal healthcare reform has not yet made clear what the exact role is for the APN; however, it does seem to offer a unique opportunity for expansion of practice. What is clear though is that APNs are satisfied with their roles in practice, and that they feel validated and valued as autonomous, independent participants in the interprofessional team. Furthermore, patients are satisfied with their services.

References

Agosta, L. J. (2009) Patient satisfaction with nurse practitioner delivered primary healthcare services. *Journal of the American Academy of Nurse Practitioner*, *21*(11): 610–617.

AACN (2011) American Association of Colleges of Nursing Master's Essentials. https://www.aacnnursing.org/Portals/0/PDFs/Publications/MastersEssentials11.pdf (Accessed 05/06/26)

American Academy of Family Practitioners (2006) *Guidelines on the Supervision of Certified Nurse Midwives, Nurse Practitioners and Doctors Assistants*. Available from: www.aafp.org.

American Academy of Nurse Practitioners (AANP) (2002) *Standards of Practice*. Available from: www.aanp.org (accessed 14/06/2011). In: S. A. Weilland, (2008) Reflections on independence in nurse practitioner practice. *Journal of the American Academy of Nurse Practitioners*. *22*(*1*): 345–352.

American Association of Colleges of Nursing (2021) *Essentials: Core Competencies for Professional Nursing Education* (revised).

American Association of Colleges of Nursing (AACN) (2011) *The Essentials of Master's Education in Nursing*. AACN: Washington DC. Available from: www.aacnnursing.org/Portals/0/PDFs/Publications/MastersEssentials11.pdf (accessed 04/06/2026).

American Nurses Association (ANA) (2007) *Public Health Nursing. Scope and Standards of Public Health Nursing*. Silver Springs, MD: American Nursing Association.

APRN Consensus Work Group and the National Council of States Boards of Nursing APRN Advisory Committee (2008) *Consensus Model for APRN Regulation: Licensure, Accreditation, Certification & Education*. Available from: www.ncsbn.org/public-files/Consensus_Model_Report.pdf (accessed 04/06/2026).

Atkins, R. and Szanton, S. (2025) Reimagining nursing education. *Stanford Social Innovation Review*. (webinar) https://ssir.org/articles/entry/reimagining-nursing-education (Accessed 04/06/226).

Avery, M. D. and Howe, C. (2007) The DNP and entry into midwifery practice: An analysis. *Journal of Midwifery & Women's Health*, *52*(1): 14–22.

Beeber, A. S., Palmer, C., Waldrop, J., Lynn, M. R. and Jones, C. B. (2019) The role of doctor nursing practice-prepared nurses in practice settings. *Nursing Outlook*, *67*(4): 354–364.

BHPR (2014) *Professional Practice Indices*. Available from www.oralhealthworkforce.org/wp-content/uploads/2016/08/DH_Professional_Practice_Index_By_State_2014.pdf (Accessed 04/06/26).

Bricker, C., Canale, M.,Hay, B., Taylor, T., Maguire, M., Remo, E., Smith, S., Johansson, M, and Morgan, H. (2022) Pandemic response: The identification of altetrnaive clinical hours to ensure advanced practice nursing students meet program requirements. *Journal of the American Association of Nurse Practitioners 34*(8): 1008–1015.

Brooten, D., Youngblut, J. M., Deatrick, J., Naylor M. and York, R. (2023) Patient problems, advanced practice nurse (APN) interventions, time and contacts among five patient groups. *Journal of Nursing Scholarship*, *35*(1): 773–779.

Chike-Harris, K., Snyder, E. and Conner, R. S. (2022). Educating APRN students about telehealth credentialing, licensing, and billing. *Journal of Nursing Education*, *61*(7): 414–446.

Cox, C., Gibbons, H. and Whiteing, N. (2010) Advanced practice in ophthalmic nursing. *Eye News Journal*, *17*(1): 17–24.

Cox, C. and Hall, A. (2007) Advanced practice role in gastrointestinal nursing. *Journal of Gastrointestinal Nursing*, *5*(4): 26–31.

De Navas-Walk, C., Proctor, B. D. and Smith, J. C. (2010) Income, Poverty and Health Insurance Coverage in the United States: 2009. Available from: www.census.gov/prod/2010pubs/p60-238.pdf (accessed 14/06/2011).

Deshefy-Longhi, T., Swartz, M. K. and Grey, M. (2008) Characterizing nurse practitioner practice by patient encounters: An APRNet study. *Journal of the American Academy of Nurse Practitioners*, *20*(5): 281–287.

Easom, A. (2005) APN and APRN are the appropriate credentials. *Nephrology Nursing Journal*, *32*(2): 86–87. Available from: http://proquest.umi.com/pqdweb?index=16&sid=1&rschmode=1&vinst=PROD&fmt=2&s (accessed 14/06/2011).

Evans, S. T. (2010) Convenient care clinics: Making a positive change in health care. *Journal of the American Academy of Nurse Practitioners*, *22*(1): 23–26.

Faris, J. A., Douglas, M. K., Maples, D. C., Berg, L. R. and Thraikill, A. (2010) Job satisfaction of advanced practice nurses in the Veterans Health Administration. *Journal of the American Academy of Nurse Practitioners*, *22*(1): 35–44.

Finkelman, A. and Kenner, C. (2007) *Teaching IOM: Implications of the Institute of Medicine Reports for Nursing Education*. 2nd Ed. Silver Springs, MD: American Nurses Association.

Fontana, J. S. (2008) The social and political forces affecting prescribing practices for chronic pain. *Journal of Professional Nursing*, *24*(1): 30–35.

Goudreau, K. A., Clark, A., Fulton, J. and Sendelbach, S. (2007) A vision of the future for clinical nurse specialists. *Clinical Nurse Specialist*, *21*(6): 310–320.

Hauer, K. E., Durning, S. J., Kernan, W. N., Fagin, M. J. and O'Sullivan, P. S. (2008) Factors associated with medical students' career choices regarding internal medicine. *Journal of the American Medical Association*, *300*(10): 1154–1164.

He, W., Sengupta, M., Velkoff, V. and DeBarros, K. (2005) *Current Population Reports: 65 + in the United States*. Washington, DC: US Census Bureau, Government Printing Office. In: J. M. Stanley, K. E. Werner and K. Apple (Eds), 2009. Positioning advanced practice registered nurses for health care reform: consensus on APRN regulation. *Journal of Professional Nursing*, *25*(6): 340–348.

Institute of Medicine (1999) *To Err Is Human*. Washington, DC: The National Academies Press.

Institute of Medicine (2001) *Crossing the Quality Chasm*. Washington, DC: The National Academies Press.

Institute of Medicine (2003a) *Priority Areas for National Action: Transforming Healthcare Quality*. Washington, DC: The National Academies Press.

Institute of Medicine (2003b) *Future of the Public's Health in the 21st Century*. Washington, DC: The National Academies Press.

Institute of Medicine (2003c) *Who will Keep the Public Healthy?* Washington, DC: The National Academies Press.

Kennedy-Malone, L., Gontraz, J., Monge, E., Harlow, S. and Boles, S. (2023) Perceived effectiveness of nursing faculty of clinical video simulation for use in nurse practitioner education. *The Journal for Nurse Practitioners. 19*(6) doi:10.1016/j.nurpra. accessed from https://pubmed.ncbi.nlm.nih.gov/37193015/ (Accessed 04/06/26.

Kleinpell, R. M., Hravnak, M., Hinch, B. and Llewellyn, J. (2008) Developing advanced practice nursing credentialing model for acute care facilities. *Nursing Administration Quarterly*, *32*(4): 279–287.

Ladak, A. and Sasinski, J. (2021) Clinical nurse specialist expands to crisis management role during COVID-19 pandemic. *Clinical Nurse Specialist*. 35(6): 291–299.

Li, Y., Wang, C., Wei, T. and Jiang, Y. (2023) The transition to advanced practice nuraing: A systematic review of qualitative studies. *International Journal of Nursing Studies 144*(5): 104525 doi: 10.1016/jnurstu 2023. 104525. www.researchgate.net/publication/370781450_The_transition_to_advanced_practice_nursing_A_systematic_review_of_qualitative_studies (Accessed 04/06/26).

McIltrot, K., Russell, N. G., Renda, S. and Fingerhood, M. (2022). Approach to advanced practice nursing student clinical during COVID-19. *Nurse Education Report Nursing . Nurs Open. 2023 Mar;10(3):1931-1935. doi: 10.1002/nop2.1404. Epub 2022 Oct 17* (Accessed 04/06/26).

Mercer Ray, M. (2008) Advanced practice registered nurse policy issues in today's health care climate. *Journal of Emergency Nursing*, *34*(6): 555–557.

Millet, C. P. (2022) *Population Health. Epidemiology for the APN. A Population Health Perspective*. Springer Publishing Co.

National Organisation of Nurse Practitioner Faculties Domains and Core Competencies of Nurse Practitioner Practice (NONPF, 2006) Available from: https://cdn.ymaws.com/www.nonpf.org/resource/resmgr/competencies/domainsandcorecomps2006.pdf (Accessed 04/06/26).

NCSBN Model Act, Revised 2021. *APRN Compact. Key Provision.*

Nursing and Midwifery Council (2005) *Annex 1 Domains of Practice and Competencies, NMC Consultation on a Proposed Framework for Post-registration Nursing*. London: NMC.

NONPF (2022) National Organisation of Nurse Practitioner Faculties Domains and Core Competencies of Nurse Practitioner Practice (2006). https://www.nonpf.org/page/NP_Role_Core_Competencies (Accessed 05/06/2026)

O'Reilly-Jacob, M., Perloff, J.,Sherafat-Kazenzadeh, R. and Flanagan, J. (2022) Nursing practitioner' perception of temporary full practice authority during a COVID-19 surge: A qualitative study. *International Journal of Nursing Studies*. 126 (104141). Doi 10.1016/j.jurstu. (Accessed 05/06/26).

Osborne, M., Rettig, A., Lindsey, A., Mathey, K., Sinnott, L. and McMahon, D. (2022) Supporting advanced practice fellowship during COVID-19. *Journal of Advanced Practice Oncology*, *13*(8): 816–821.

Partin, B. (2009) APRN/Physician collaboration: A call to action. *Nurse Practitioner*, *34*(1): 6. Available from: http://proquest.umi.com/pqdweb?index=1&sid=1&srchmode=1&vinst=PROD&fmt=2&st (Accessed 16/03/2010).

Phillips (2010) 22nd Annual Legislative Update: Regulatory and legislative successes of ARPNs. *The Nurse Practitioner*, *35*(1): 24–47. www.tnpj.com.

Public Health Law 111–148 (2011). Available from: www.gpo.gov/fdsys/pkg/PLAW-111publ148/pdf/PLAW-111publ148.pdf (Accessed 14/06/2011).

Raymond, L., Castonquay, A., Doyon, O. and Pare, G. (2022) Nurse practitioner' involvement and experience with AI-based health technologies: A systematic review. *Applied Nursing Research* 66, 151604. www.sciencedirect.com/science/article/abs/pii/S0897189722000465 (Accessed 05/06/26).

Royal College of Nursing ((2011) *Advanced Nurse Practitioners – An RCN Guide to the Advanced Nurse Practitioner Role, Competences and Programme Accreditation.* Available from: https://www.google.com/search?q=Royal+College+of+Nursing+%282010a%29+%282011%29Advanced+Nurse+Practitioners+%E2%80%93+An+RCN+Guide+to+the+Advanced+Nurse+Practitioner+Role%2C+Competences+and+Programme+Accreditation&oq=Royal+College+of+Nursing+%282010a%29+%282011%29Advanced+Nurse+Practitioners+%E2%80%93+An+RCN+Guide+to+the+Advanced+Nurse+Practitioner+Role%2C+Competences+and+Programme+Accreditation&gs_lcrp=EgZjaHJvbWUyBggAEEUYOdIBBzkxMmowajSoAgCwAgA&sourceid=chrome&ie=UTF-8 (Accessed 05/06/26)

Sonney, J. and Peck, J. J. (2023). The cost of caring during COVID-19: A clarion call to action to support the paediatric advanced practice nursing workforce. *Journal of Paediatric Health Care.37*(6): pp 658–672. https://pubmed.ncbi.nlm.nih.gov/37725029/ (Accessed 05/06/26).

Stanley, J. M., Werner, K. E. and Apple, K. (2009) Positioning advanced practice registered nurses for health care reform: Consensus on APRN regulation. *Journal of Professional Nursing, 25*(6): 340–348.

Stewart, J. G., McNulty, R. M., Quinn Griffin, A. T. and Fitzpatrick, J. J. (2010) Psychological empowerment and structural empowerment among nurse practitioners. *Journal of the American Academy of Nurse Practitioners, 22*(1): 27–34.

Tuite, P. K. and George, E. L. (2010) The role of the clinical nurse specialist in facilitating evidence-based practice within a university setting. *Critical Care Nursing Quarterly, 33*(2): 117–125.

Upvall, M. J. and Ptachcinski, R. J. (2007) The journey to the DNP programme and beyond: What we can learn from pharmacy? *Journal of Professional Nursing, 23*(5): 316–321.

Vasquez, B. A., Moreno-Lacalle, R., Soriano, G. P., Juntasoopeepun, P. and Loscin, R. C. (2023) Technological Machines and Artificial Intelligence in Nursing Practice. *Nursing & Health Sciences: Wiley. 25*(3): pp 474–481. https://pubmed.ncbi.nlm.nih.gov/37332058/ (Accessed 05/06/2026).

Watts, S., Gee, J., O'Day, M. E., Schaub, K., Lawrence, R., Aron, D. and Kirsh, S. (2009) Nurse practitioner-led multidisciplinary teams to improve chronic illness care: The unique strengths of nurse practitioners applied to shared medical appointments/group visits. *Journal of the American Academy of Nurse Practitioners, 21*(3): 167–172. https://onlinelibrary.wiley.com/doi/abs/10.1111/j.1745-7599.2008.00379.x (Accessed 05/06/26)

Weilland, A. (2008) Reflections on independence in nurse practitioner practice. *Journal of the American Academy of Nurse Practitioners, 221*(7): 345–352. (Accessed 24/03/2011).

Wood, E., King, R., Taylor, B., Roberston, S., Senek, M., Tod, A. and Ryan, T. (2022) Moral distress in advanced practice nurses during the COVID-19 pandemic. *Nursing Standard,* 11:44–50.

PART 3

Leadership

The professional role

CHAPTER 8

Professionalism in advanced practice

The professional role

Carol L. Cox

Introduction

Professionalism is defined as 'the conduct, aims, or qualities that characterise or mark a profession or a professional person' (Merriam-Webster, 2003; 2022). However, more recent understandings and interpretations of professionalism also include modern perspectives like authenticity, cultural awareness and emotional intelligence (Merriam-Webster, 2022). 'In assuming a professional role, one conforms to the technical or ethical standards of a profession exhibiting a courteous, conscientious and generally businesslike manner in the workplace' (Merriam-Webster, 2003:991). This quote can be understood to mean a professional has the skill and discernment to make good judgements whilst incorporating courteous behaviour that is expected from a person who has been educated and trained in their profession. In other words, to do their job well.

According to Brehm et al. (2006), the concept of professionalism is multifaceted. Professionalism may be divided into three components or categories which are: professional parameters (knowledge and skills), professional behaviours (conduct and interaction) and professional responsibilities (service and ethics) (Wood, 2025; Bossers et al., 1999). Professional parameters include legal and ethical issues whilst professional behaviours are related to discipline-related knowledge and skills, relationships with clients and colleagues in which collaboration and collegiality become essential components and an acceptable appearance and attitude. Professionalism is situational and adaptive (Wood, 2025; Cao et al., 2023). Finally professional responsibilities relate to a responsibility to one's profession, to oneself, to clients, to employers and to the community. Individuals must develop the full spectrum of characteristics, attitudes and behaviours including a life-long commitment to professionalism if one is to be regarded

DOI: 10.4324/9781003609049-12

as a professional (Tan and Chin, 2023; Wood, 2025; Brehm et al., 2006; Hammer et al., 2003).

Learning outcomes

At the conclusion of this chapter, you will be able to:

- Describe the elements of professionalism associated with clinical/direct care advanced practice
- Discuss professionalism in relation to leadership and collaborative advanced practice
- Relate professionalism to improving quality and developing advanced practice
- Formulate plans for developing self and others at an advanced practice level

Background

The Council for Healthcare Regulatory Excellence (CHRE, 2009) confirmed the need for a nationally agreed set of standards for advanced-level practice in nursing. Since that event it has been recognised that all professions involved in direct care delivery working at an advanced level of practice, regardless of the area of practice, setting or client group, should be practising to the same level of standards. In November 2010, the Department of Health (DoH) for England under the auspices of the Chief Nursing Officer for England, Dame Christine Beasley, published its definitive position statement on Advanced Level Nursing. In the document it is indicated that the purpose of the statement is to 'improve understanding of advanced level practice, and will act as an aid to assist practitioners, commissioners, educators, service and workforce planners achieve their aim of building services focused on improving outcomes and experiences for patients' (DoH, 2010:2). The position statement is intended to be used as a benchmark that will enhance patient safety and the delivery of high-quality care. Without question, this document is an indication of standards associated with professionalism. In this chapter the essential elements associated with professionalism at an advanced practice level will be addressed. These elements are explicated in the DoH (2010) position statement and for the purpose of this chapter will be associated with all healthcare professions involved in the delivery of care to patients. The nationally agreed elements of advanced practice are described under four themes. These themes are: Clinical/direct care practice; Leadership and collaborative practice; Improving quality and developing practice; and Developing self and others (DoH, 2010:5).

Linked to each theme are elements associated with advanced practice. These elements should be regarded as a minimum threshold that demonstrates the essential attributes of professionalism. In relation to professionalism, professionalism involves respect for patients and coworkers, knowledge of discipline, accountability, flexibility, trustworthiness, ethical behaviour, teamwork, confidentiality, honesty and reliability (Parastesh et al., 2025; Wood, 2025; Cao and Song, 2023; NMC, 2023; Brehm at al., 2006). Clarification of these elements involves:

- **Knowledge of Discipline:** Maintaining a deep and current understanding of one's specific field of practice.

- **Accountability:** Taking ownership of actions, decisions and outcomes related to patient care and professional responsibilities.
- **Flexibility:** Adapting to changing clinical situations, patient needs and healthcare environments.
- **Trustworthiness:** Acting in a reliable and consistent manner that inspires confidence from patients, families and colleagues.
- **Ethical Behaviour:** Adhering to established ethical principles and professional codes of conduct.
- **Teamwork:** Collaborating effectively with interdisciplinary teams to provide coordinated and comprehensive care.
- **Confidentiality:** Protecting patient information and maintaining privacy in accordance with legal and ethical standards.
- **Honesty:** Being truthful in all professional interactions, documentation and communication.
- **Reliability:** Consistently meeting obligations and commitments, ensuring dependable presence and performance in the practice setting.

These elements, derived from foundational concepts of professionalism, form the core attributes expected of individuals engaged in advanced practice roles. Furthermore, in accordance with the position statement on advanced practice, it can be seen that professionalism is underpinned by the assumptions that all healthcare professionals: take personal responsibility for their actions and omissions and fully recognise their personal accountability; can make sound decisions about their ongoing personal and professional development; practice within the scope of their personal professional competence and extend this scope as appropriate; delegate aspects of care to others and accept responsibility and accountability for such delegation; work harmoniously and effectively with colleagues, patients and clients and their carers, families and friends (Cao and Song, 2023; Elksas et al., 2021; Hasan et al., 2016; Fantahun et al., 2014). Society expects these individuals to conduct themselves within an ethical framework based upon respect for the well-being and safety of patients and clients (Parastesh et al, 2025; Palmer et al., 2024; Shohani and Zamanzadeh, 2017; DoH, 2010:5). The advanced practice nurse possesses a sense of oneself, and this sense is carried over into relationships with others (Bobek et al., 2025). Overall, these senses are influenced by the characteristics, norms and values of the nursing discipline, resulting in individual thinking and acting in the clinical arena (Bobek et al., 2025).

Professionalism in advanced clinical practice

Professionalism can be readily recognised in the definition of advanced-level nursing published by the Department of Health (DoH, 2010). According to the Department of Health (DoH, 2010:7), at an advanced practice level, the healthcare professional is 'deeply involved in promoting public health and well-being.' These professionals 'understand the implications of the social, economic and political context of healthcare and their professional and clinical judgement are demonstrated in the Expert nature of their practice and depth of their knowledge' (DoH, 2010:7). Furthermore, patients, clients and other professionals acknowledge their highly developed and extensive knowledge in areas such as 'diagnostics, therapeutics, biological, social and epidemiological sciences and pharmacology and their enhanced skills in consultation and clinical decision-making' (DoH, 2010:7). Healthcare professionals working at an advanced practice level use 'complex reasoning, critical thinking, reflection and analysis to inform their assessment, clinical judgements and decisions. They can apply knowledge and skills to a broad range of clinically and professionally challenging and complex situations' (DoH, 2010:7). These attributes are clearly identified in research literature published nationally and internationally (Tan and Chin, 2023; Cao and Song, 2023; Palmer et al., 2023)

The Nursing and Midwifery Council (NMC, 2010:1) produced a consultation document on advanced practice for nurses in 2005 in which it indicated that these nurses:

- Take a comprehensive patient history
- Carry out physical examinations
- Use their expert knowledge and clinical judgement to identify the potential diagnosis
- Refer patients for investigations where appropriate
- Make a final diagnosis
- Decide on and carry out treatment, including the prescribing of medicines, or refer patients to an appropriate specialist
- Use their extensive practice experience to plan and provide skilled and competent care to meet patients' health and social care needs, involving other members of the healthcare team as appropriate
- Ensure the provision of continuity of care including follow-up visits
- Assess and evaluate, with patients, the effectiveness of the treatment and care provided and make changes as needed
- Work independently, although often as part of a healthcare team
- Provide leadership
- Make sure that each patient's treatment and care is based on best practice

Reflecting back to February 2006, it was agreed that these were the definitive activities of the advanced nurse practitioner. In addition, it indicated that 'Advanced nurse practitioners are highly experienced and educated members of the care team who are able to diagnose and treat your health care needs or refer you to an appropriate specialist if needed' (NMC, 2010:1). Aspects of these activities and their definition of the advanced nurse practitioner can be seen as defining characteristics of all advanced practitioners in relation to attributes of professionalism in practice. Table 8.1 shows the NMC (2010) competencies associated with the practice element of the professional role that was originally published in 2005. Subsequently, it must be acknowledged that the Nuffield Trust, following extensive research, published an Independent Report on the regulation of advanced practice in nursing and midwifery in which these definitive activities were recognised (Palmer et al., 2024).

It is apparent from the competencies listed in Table 8.1 that there is a blending of clinical practice, leadership, education and research into the clinical role. The advanced healthcare practitioner is functioning as a co-ordinator, consultant, coach, advocate, administrator, educator, researcher, role model and leader in addition to providing direct patient care (Tan and Chin, 2023 Palmer, 2024).

Table 8.1 Nursing and Midwifery Council Competencies in the Professional Role Related to Practice

Competencies
Develops and implements the advanced nurse practitioner role
1 Uses evidence and research to implement the role.
2 Functions in a variety of role dimensions: healthcare provider, coordinator, consultant, educator, coach, advocate, administrator, researcher, role model and leader.
3 Interprets and markets the role to the public, legislators, policy-makers and other healthcare professions.
Directs care
1 Prioritises, coordinates and meets multiple needs for culturally diverse patients.
2 Uses sound judgement in assessing conflicting priorities and needs.
3 Builds and maintains a therapeutic team to provide optimum therapy.
4 Obtains specialist and referral care for patients while remaining the primary care provider.
5 Acts as an advocate for the patient to ensure health needs are met consistent with patients' wishes.
6 Consults with other healthcare providers and public/independent agencies.
7 Incorporates current technology appropriately in care delivery.
8 Uses information systems to support decision-making and to improve care.

Source: NMC (2025a); NMC (2010:17 'Consultation Document').

Before delineating the competencies in Table 8.1, Nursing and Midwifery Council Competencies in the Professional Role Related to Practice, (NMC, 2010), it is useful to review the NMC (2025) perspective on advanced-level practice. The NMC (2025a, b; NMC, 2023) views advanced practice as a level of expert practice, requiring postgraduate education, operating with high autonomy and integrating the 'four pillars': clinical practice, leadership, education and research, to manage complex care across settings. It's about expertise, not just a title, involving complex decision-making, risk management and driving improvements, often underpinned by master's-level learning (Level 7).

Learning the professional role

Professionalism is informally learned through role modelling by other professionals, instructors and preceptors. What is critical within the process of learning a professional role is assimilation of the values and behaviours associated with the discipline being acquired. Health professionals should be taught to coordinate, collaborate and communicate with one another in interdisciplinary teams so that appropriate clinical decisions are made and ethical dilemmas are solved (Bobek et al., 2025; Brehm et al., 2006; Institute of Medicine, Committee on Quality of Health Care in America, 2001; Cloonan et al., 1999). To achieve this, it involves the integration of discipline-specific knowledge, skills and perspectives. In so doing, optimal patient care that encompasses the expertise of each health professional can be delivered (Brehm et al., 2006; Brennan, 2002). Interdisciplinary learning opportunities enhance understanding and appreciation of one's profession and its potential contributions to the healthcare team.

Activity 1

Identify aspects of your practice in which you have learned to practise at an advanced practice level through the role modelling of others.

Answer the following questions:

- How do you function as a role model for others?
- Do you role model in the same way as your instructors and preceptors have role modelled for you?
- What aspects of role modelling come easily to you?

What aspects of role modelling are difficult for you and how can you overcome these difficulties?

Tip for helping others learn

The goals of learning are to stress the importance of professionalism in the clinical environment, to provide information in relation to the various health disciplines and interdisciplinary teams that are involved in healthcare. One good way to learn about what is appropriate is to consider what is not appropriate. This can be initiated through role play in which clinically based scenarios are enacted in which non-professional behaviours, skills and attitudes are reviewed. Field experience provides opportunities to gain insight into the roles and responsibilities of other health professionals. Here, professional traits and behaviours can be observed in a natural setting. The learner can consider how their own discipline might contribute to care in the context in which healthcare is being delivered.

Professionalism in relation to leadership and collaborative advanced practice

Leadership and collaboration

Collaborating with others sounds easy on the face of it. However, with diverse interests in practice disciplines and competing demands for the patient's or client's healthcare regimen it is possible to come into conflict regarding the best plan of care for the patient/client. Plochg et al. (2009:2) state that 'As the status of medical work is, at least in part, competitive, professional- ization is linked to the pursuit of internal control over medical work and outperforming rival specialities.' Brennan (2002) and Plochg et al. (2009) indicate that a commitment must be made to working with others to ensure that healthcare teams working within the healthcare environment produce the best possible outcomes for patients. This means taking up the banner to lead systematic analyses of quality care and working with others to develop better methods of care (Hargreaves and O'Connor, 2025; Katz et al, 2007). According to the Department of Health (2010) and the NMC (2023) this involves providing consultancy services to one's own and other professions in relation to therapeutic interventions and practice and service development. It also means working 'across professional, organisational and system boundaries and proactively developing and sustaining new partnerships and networks to influence and improve health, outcomes and healthcare delivery systems' (DoH, 2010:10). Within the context of leadership, the Department of Health (2010) has also been clear that the advanced practice practitioner engages stakeholders and uses high-level negotiating and influencing skills to develop and improve practice. Part of this can come about through recognition of a need for change (Shiriag et al., 2025). However, moving forward to generating practice innovations and then leading on practice and service redesign solutions that meet the needs of patients/clients and the service in better ways sometimes means changing the perspective on relationships between doctors, managers and other healthcare clinicians. The perspective is changed to ensure that the improvements recommended are based on careful research and data that have been mediated by continuous quality improvement methods (Tan and Chin, 2023; Brennan, 2002). Generating practice innovations and leading on practice and service redesign are essential components of the advanced practice practitioner's remit over the past two decades. Healthcare reform has brought about a change in the structure of healthcare, both in the primary care and secondary care sectors. Considerable progress has been made in making healthcare more accessible to patients and moving healthcare management to the control of non-doctor health system managers (Taylor, 1996). This places the advanced practice practitioner in an ideal position to manage a multidisciplinary healthcare team. Leading a multidisciplinary healthcare team requires considerable tact, discretionary and experiential expertise and is an inherent component of clinical practice (Tan and Chin, 2023; Plochg et al., 2009). Expertise and knowledge are required to navigate patients through systems, and ensure that patients experience not only better health outcomes but also that costs associated with delivering healthcare are controlled effectively. Knowledge of health policy and how systems relate between the primary and secondary care sectors is invaluable. Additionally active involvement in one's professional organisation/college can provide much-needed guidance and support professionals undertaking leadership positions. Table 8.2 (NMC, 2010), Nursing and

Table 8.2 Nursing and Midwifery Council Competencies in the Professional Role Related to Leadership

Competencies
Provides leadership
1 Is actively involved in a professional association.
2 Evaluates implications of contemporary health policy on healthcare providers and consumers.
3 Participates in legislative and policy-making activities that influence an advanced level of nursing practice and the health of communities.
4 Advocates for access to quality, cost-effective healthcare.
5 Evaluates the relationship between community/public health issues and social problems as they impact on the healthcare of patients (poverty, literacy, violence, etc.).
6 Actively engages in continuous professional development and maintains a suitable record of this development.

Source: NMC (2010:17 'Consultation Document').

Activity 2

Consider your involvement in the healthcare team. Are you influencing change? Are you leading a team? If 'no' is your response, what do you need to do to increase the leadership components of your professional role?

Construct a plan of action for a healthcare innovation that you think requires introduction in your healthcare setting. How feasible is it to implement this plan of action? What negotiating skills do you need to bring about introduction of the innovation?

Midwifery Council Competencies in the Professional Role Related to Practice, shows the NMC (NMC, 2025a, b; NMC, 2010) competencies associated with the leadership element of the professional role that were originally published in 2005.

Improving quality, developing practice, self and others
Autonomous practice, self-direction and self-regulation

In June 2025, the NMC (NMC, 2025a) articulated its principles for advanced practice. The principles intend to bring clarity and consistency to advanced practice across the UK (NMC, 2025a). The principles will:

For the public: they will help patients and people who use services to understand the role of an advanced practitioner, including a definition that is clearly understood by members of the public.

For professionals: they will help professionals deliver consistent, high-quality, safe and effective delivery of care by setting clear expectations for advanced practice nursing and midwifery.

For employers: they will help employers to develop and sustain systems in which advanced practice can thrive – for example in workforce, education, support, continuing professional development (CPD) and governance planning.

Essential components of professionalism within the context of advanced practice include autonomous practice, self- direction, self-regulation and proactive involvement in the development of strategies and the undertaking of activities that monitor and improve the quality of healthcare and the effectiveness of one's own and others' practice (CMS. Gov., 2025; NMC, 2025 a, b; DoH, 2010). The aim of professional self-regulation is to make individual practitioners more accountable to their peers (NMC, 2025a; van Herk et al., 2001; Klein, 2013). Clinical autonomy can be considered the core of professional autonomy (Mahon, 2015; van Herk et al., 2001). Clnical or technical autonomy is defined as the right of the profession to set its own standards and control clinical performance (Elston and Bury, 1991). As an autonomous advanced practice practitioner, the healthcare professional continually assesses and monitors risk in relation to their own and others' practice and challenges others about wider risk factors (Mahon, 2015; DoH, 2010). These individuals 'plan and seize opportunities to generate and apply new knowledge to their own and others' practice in structured ways which are capable of evaluation' (DoH, 2010:11) through clinical audit and other mechanisms. Brennan (2002), Katz et al. (2007) and Plochg et al. (2009). There is a new civic professionalism that is calling for systematic quality measurement and improvement. Brennan (2002:976) further indicates that an

> observer of the past 20 years of our health system might remark that professionalism has been eclipsed somewhat as a source of reform for health care institutions ... by the market ... and regulatory approaches sponsored by the government. The mandates of professional obligations are rarely used (anymore) to justify reform.

However, this has not been the case traditionally, nor should it be the only route recognised as providing the platform for quality care. The healthcare professions are defined as occupations controlling specific knowledge within their disciplines and hence possessing specific activities in commerce (Lebovits et al., 1997; Brennan, 2002) that have been and are held to higher expectations by the public. As such there is a professional obligation to take seriously the mandate of promoting quality care. The Department of Health (2010) indicates that advanced practice practitioners 'continually evaluate and audit the practice of self and others at individual and systems levels, selecting and applying valid and reliable approaches and methods which are appropriate to needs and context, and acting on the findings' (DoH, 2010:10). They further 'strive constantly to improve practice and health outcomes so that they are consistent with or better than national and international standards through initiating, facilitating and leading change at individual, team, organisational and system levels' (DoH, 2010:10). It may be argued that professionalism can be considered a platform for reform of the healthcare system and a means of delivering high-quality care. It may also be argued that professionalism should be understood as an ideology of social reform (Brennan, 2002; McGlynn and Brook, 2001). As an alternative to market demand and government regulatory approaches, professionalism can infuse social responsibility (Sullivan, 1999) into the healthcare system. In this perspective advanced practice practitioners must be seen as advocates for their patients/clients and carers as well. As responsible autonomous practitioners they must advocate for and on behalf of the community of patients and their interests.

Civic professionalism

The principles underlying civic professionalism have derived from traditional professional values and extend the accountability of advanced practice to a social contract with the public. In this model, under the direction of the advanced practice practitioner, patients take an active role in shaping healthcare delivery (Katz et al., 2007). Brennan (2002:979) indicates that 'Civic professionalism's movement from individual obligation to social obligation can help provide the intellectual base for treating health as a system.' Civic professionalism in relation to quality improvements mandates a team effort in today's healthcare organisations.

The Department of Health (2010:9) was clear in 2010 and now that as autonomous and self-directed professionals, advanced practice practitioners 'identify and implement systems to promote their contribution and demonstrate the impact of advanced level practice to the healthcare team and the wider health and social care sector'. Therefore, there must be a commitment to professional competence, a commitment to lifelong learning through continuous professional development and recertification and a commitment to establishing trust with patients and fostering honesty with patients;

Tip regarding civic professionalism

Society at large defines quality in terms of the healthcare organisation promoting health and preventing error. Your professional role as an advanced practice practitioner is to maintain integrity, compassion, excellence, continuous quality improvement and working in partnership with the healthcare team.

particularly when errors occur in healthcare (Bobek et al., 2025; Katz et al., 2007). In relation to civic professional norms, there is a requirement that patients be informed promptly so that a trusting relationship is maintained between the advanced practice practitioner and the patient/client and their carers. In addition, it is essential that a commitment to improving the quality of care is undertaken. Professionalism mandates that the advanced practice practitioner maintains their clinical competence and works with other professionals to ensure that the best possible outcomes are produced for patients within the context of all healthcare settings – be it primary, secondary or tertiary care. In the United Kingdom and in the United States of America as well as many other countries there is a Patient Charter indicating that quality care will be provided and maintained. Additionally, in consideration of professionalism, as advanced practice practitioners there is an obligation to act as role models, to actively participate in interdisciplinary teams, to actively use data and to promote the use of evidence-based practice (NMC, 2025a; NMC 2025b). Poor-quality care must be reported when it occurs, and appropriate use of quality systems must be utilised to prevent inappropriate care (Katz et al., 2007). Professionalism represents a contract between highly trained professionals and the public (Cao et al., 2023; Brennan, 2002). This contract creates special responsibilities; the most critical being promoting quality of care. Modern quality improvement requires team effort. This means working together to place patient welfare at his or her highest value (NMC 2025b; Parastesh et al., 2025; Brennan, 2002) and to enhance the patient experience. Quality of care is impacted and professionalism is lost in instances of complacency, arrogance, inability to self-regulate, a 'head in the sand' syndrome and poor leadership (Koornhof, 2025; Hughes, 2006). Factors associated with a decline in professionalism include a perspective of the locus of control over practice being external to the individual and a loss of discretion (Harrison and Ahmad, 2000).

Activity 3

Consider how you can be involved in developing systems of better quality when your time is limited, due to the expansive number of patients you are responsible for managing.

Assessment of professionalism

Assessment of professionalism incorporates measuring observable behaviours (conduct, competence, communication, ethics, appearance, reliability) and underlying values (integrity, empathy, accountability) through multi-faceted methods like 360-degree feedback, observed clinical encounters, self-assessments and structured tools. The tools developed must recognise the complex, context-dependent construct requiring longitudinal evaluation, not just a single entity. Assessment combines external actions with internal

Tip about patient welfare

As professionals, advanced practice practitioners place patient welfare as their highest value.

principles, making objective measurement challenging but crucial, especially in fields like healthcare (Goldie, 2013). Measuring professionalism is a difficult process. According to Goldie (2013) and Hodges et al. (2009) there is no specific method that has emerged as the definitive means of assessing professionalism. Literature reviews demonstrate a lack of current evidence when measuring attitudes related to professionalism in medical and other healthcare professions' educational processes. In medical education the different methods of assessing professionalism have been proposed (Parastesh et al., 2025; Lynch et al., 2004). Outside of medical education the landscape for assessing professionalism becomes more bereft. Generally, competency assessment frameworks are espoused as a mechanism for assessing aspects of professionalism (Goldie, 2013; Plochg et al., 2009; Ruth et al., 2008; Katz et al., 2007); however, these frameworks lack specifics and are external mechanisms with limited impact on changing behaviour. A sign of professionalism is recognition of lapses in professional judgement. However, determining the best method of assessing recognition and subsequent professionalism can be tortuous. Identification of the responsibilities of the healthcare professional is a necessary step in the process of assessment and remediation (Welbourn and Theodore, 2010). Reflection has been shown to be highly important in the development of professional behaviours (Sherwood, 2024; Johns, 2010; Hodges et al., 2009). Lapses in professional judgement can be explored through reflection in practice; thus, leading to significant development of professional behaviour.

When advanced practice practitioners recognise through reflection that there has been a lapse in professional judgement and demonstrate guilt and remorse for their actions there is potential for remedial action. They can acknowledge a lack of knowledge and skill. This action is termed 'acceptance' (Hodges et al., 2009). Denial of a fault in themselves is associated with feelings of the situation being out of their control. This action is termed 'rejection' (Hodges et al., 2009) and can have serious consequences in terms of patient health outcomes. Reporting and reflecting is a sign of maturity in the professional. Reporting and reflecting demonstrate acceptance. Reflection provides a strong platform from which lapses in professional behaviour can be improved and promotes positive changes. The absence of reflection and/or the inability to respond adequately to events is an indicator of unprofessional behaviour (Sherwood, 2024; Hodges et al., 2009). 'Report and Reflect' (Hodges et al., 2009:4) is a system of incident reporting and is a recognised mechanism for individuals to use within the context of their professional practice.

Activity 4

Critical incident reports are enhanced when combined with reflection (Hodges et al., 2009). How would you report and reflect on a critical incident that has occurred in your practice? Can you indicate an incident of 'acceptance?' Can you indicate an incident that was an occasion of 'rejection?' If the incident was one of 'rejection,' how would you, following reflection, address this incident now?

Commitment to lifelong learning

> Academic courses and seminars that require socialization and collaboration across disciplines should address professionalism, confidence in discipline specific knowledge and skills, and respect for the actual and potential contributions of the participating disciplines to optimal health care. Small group activities are effective teaching strategies that emphasise the importance of collaboration, collegiality, professionalism, decision making, and problem solving among team members.
>
> (Bobek et al., 2025; Hargreaves and O'Connor, 2025; Brehm et al., 2006:5)

To promote learning about how to collaborate across disciplines those who act as role models, instructors and preceptors must be cognisant of their own professional values and beliefs as well as those from other disciplines. They must be open and honest in their communication of their professional knowledge, skills and attitudes to those learning from them (Bobek et al, 2025; Brehm et al., 2006; Brennan, 2002; Glen, 1999). According to Sherwood (2024)

> Knowledge development to guide evidence-informed practice is a cornerstone of nursing as a practice-based discipline. The emphasis on empirical knowledge development overshadows other ways of knowledge development – personal, aesthetic, and ethical. Technical, objective knowledge development is more dominant than knowledge development for delivering holistic, person-centred care. Personal, aesthetic, and ethical ways of knowing are essential factors in satisfying work environments, patient satisfaction, and nurse retention.
>
> (Sherwood, 2024: 399)

In view of this perspective, learning must be lifelong, incorporating personal, aestietic and ethical ways of knowing in order to maintain the knowledge and skills necessary to practise at an advanced level within an ever-changing healthcare environment.

Activity 5

Consider how your professional developments are being addressed. Are you undertaking academic courses that develop or enhance your advanced practice knowledge and skills?

Tip regarding the maintenance of your professional registration

Most regulatory bodies (e.g., the NMC, the Healthcare Professions Council and the State Boards of Nursing) require thorough on-going continuous professional development through certificate and recertification programmes. Re-examination of practice is essential for validation of competent professional practice.

Indicate how you will engage others in clinical seminars designed to promote patients' health and well-being.

According to the Department of Health (2010), the learning and development requirements of healthcare professionals at an advanced practice level should be 'identified and supported through individual performance review, appraisal and revalidation requirements on an ongoing basis and alongside a robust clinical supervision framework' (DoH, 2010:6). Part of professionalism is the responsibility to continuously assess and develop one's practice.

Protecting the public

> Maintaining and improving standards of service and care are central to professionalism in health care. The origins of the bodies that now represent and regulate medicine, nursing, pharmacy, and other professions in the health care sector are closely related to the need to protect the public from 'quackery' and the excesses of competition. This is appropriate in a service where users – patients are often profoundly vulnerable.
>
> (Taylor, 1996:312)

Although this statement was written in 1996, it has resonance for advanced practice practitioners today. There have been a plethora of papers and standards of practice (refer to the Health Professions Council and the NMC Standards of Practice as examples) written to protect the public from potential harm that can occur in the healthcare system (NMC, 2025a; NMC 2025b). There is also a plethora of quality measures instituted in the healthcare system. These strong institutional structures underpin healthcare professionalism (Taylor, 1996). However, they do not substitute for the ethical values and beliefs that every advanced practice practitioner should embrace as a fundamental of their professionalism. As advocates for patients, the advanced practice practitioner has a responsibility to work towards eliminating neglect and inadequate care. Much of this can be accomplished as indicated previously in this chapter. Primarily this is accomplished by working effectively with one's clinical colleagues in the interests of patients (Ruth et al., 2008). By emphasising prevention and health promotion, the well-being of patients can be enhanced. By working effectively – proactively within the healthcare team – potential is increased to ameliorate social health problems. As a professional engaging in advanced practice, there is a moral obligation to respect patients as people, to encourage patients' involvement in the delivery of care and to ensure that their privacy and dignity are maintained (Galletta et al, 2022).

Conclusion

The increasing complexity of care, coordination of multiple patient needs and delivery of care across clinical environments mean that professionalism is an essential ingredient for positive clinical outcomes. Professionalism incorporates attributes such as respect for patients and coworkers, knowledge of discipline, technological skill, accountability, flexibility, trustworthiness, ethical behaviour, teamwork, confidentiality, honesty and reliability. Teamwork amongst disciplines should be stressed to ease the transition from a basic professional role to an advanced practice professional role. This endeavour will enhance the advanced practice practitioner's effectiveness as a member of the healthcare team.

Although the NMC does not currently specifically regulate advanced practice in nursing and midwifery, it indicates that *The Code* (NMC, 2024), which refers to professional standards for nurses, midwives and nursing associates in the UK, governs all nursing and midwifery practitioners and that advanced practice is dependent upon the nurse's or midwife's knowledge and skills. The level of professionalism the nurse demonstrates authenticates their position as an advanced practice nurse. This chapter has indicated that as professionals, one must report poor quality of care when it occurs. Advanced practice nurses must advocate for the use of appropriate systems in all areas where healthcare is provided. Finally, as an advanced practice practitioner one must actively promote patient and carer involvement in the development, delivery and evaluation of care.

References

Bobek, H., Lee, M., Roll, K., Linder, S., Shihabuddin, C. and Sharpe, E. (2025) Promoting professionalism for nurse practitioner students for clinical success. *The Journal for Nurse Practitioners*, 21(3): 105318.

Bossers, A., Kernaghan, J., Hodgins, L., Merla, L., O'Connor, C. and Van Kessel, M. (1999) Defining and developing professionalism. *Canadian Journal of Occupational Therapy*, 66(3): 16–21.

Brehm, B., Breen, P., Brown, B., Long, L., Smith, R., Wall, A. and Warren, N. (2006) Instructional design and assessment: An interdisciplinary approach to introducing professionalism. *American Journal of Pharmaceutical Education*, 70(4): 1–5.

Brennan, R. (2002) Physicians' professional responsibility to improve the quality of care. *Academic Medicine*, 77(10): 973–980.

Cao, H., Song, Y., Wu, Y. et al. (2023) What is nursing professionalism? a concept analysis. *BMC Nursing*, 22(1): 34, 10.1186/s12912-022-01161-0 (accessed 1/6/2026).

CHRE (2009) Advanced Practice: Report to the four UK Health Departments. Unique ID 17-2008. Healthcare Regulatory Excellence. Available from: https://www.professionalstandards.org.uk/sites/default/files/attachments/advanced-practice-2009.pdf (accessed 07/06/2026).

Cloonan, P., David, F. and Burnett, C. (1999) Interdisciplinary education in clinical ethics: a work in progress. *Holistic Nurse Practitioner*, 13(2): 12–19.

CMS. Gov. (2025) CMS Quality Reporting and Value-Based Programs and Initiatives. https://mmshub.cms.gov/about-quality/quality-at-CMS/quality/programs (July 2025) (accessed 7/06/2026).

DoH (2010) Advanced Level Nursing: A Position Statement. Department of Health, 403775, 10 November 2010. London: Produced by COI for the Department of Health. Available from: www.dh.gov.uk/publications (accessed 10/01/11).

Elksas E., Abd El Rahman R. and Hassan A.N. (2021) Developing an instrument for measuring bachelor's degree nursing professionalism. *Journal of Research in Nursing*, 8(1): 376–389. www.noveltyjournals.com (accessed 1/6/2026).

Elston, M. and Bury, M. (1991) The politics of professional power, medicine in a changing health service, in Gabe, J., Calnan, M. (Eds), *The Sociology of the Heatlh Service*. London: Routledge.

Fantahun A., Demessie A., Gebrekirstos K., Zemene A. and Ga Y. (2014) A cross-sectional study on factors influencing professionalism in nursing among nurses in Mekelle public hospitals, North Ethiopia. *BMC Nursing*, 13(1): 10. doi: 10.1186/1472-6955-13-10.

Galletta, M., Piazza, M., Meloni, S., Chessa, E., Piras, I, Arnetz, J. and D'Aloja, E. (2022) Patient involvement in shared decision making: do patients rate physicians and nurses differently? *International Journal of Environmental Research and Public Health*, 19(21): 14229. doi: 10.3390/ijerph192114229 (accessed 1/10/2026).

Glen, S. (1999) Educating for interprofessional collaboration: teaching about values. *Nursing Ethics*, 6(3): 202–213.

Goldie, J. (2013) Assessment of Professionalism: a consolidation of current thinking. *Medical Teacher*, 35(2): e952–e956. https://pubmed.ncbi.nlm.nih.gov/22938675/ (accessed 1/11/2026).

Hammer, D., Berger, B. and Beadsley, R. (2003) Student professionalism. *American Journal of Pharmaceutical Education*, 67(3): 1–29.

Hargreaves, A. and O'Connor, M. (2025) *Collaborative Professionalism, When Teaching Together Means Learning for All*. Sage, CQ Press Books, Thousand Oaks, California.

Harrison, S. and Ahmad, W. (2000) Medical autonomy and the UK state 1975 to 2025. *Sociology* 34(1): 129–146.

Hasan Doost F., Moghadas T., Momeni M. and Rafiei H. Factors influencing professionalism: a cross-sectional study among Iranian registered nurses. *IOSR Journal of Nursing and Health Science*, 5(3): 47–49. doi: 10.9790/7388-0603024749.

Hodges, D., McLachlan, J. and Finn, G. (2009) Exploring reflective 'critical incident' documentation of professionalism lapses in medical undergraduate setting. *BMC Medical Education*, 9(44): 1–5.

Hughes, G. (2006) Medical professionalism in the 21st century; how do we stack up? *Journal of Emergency Medicine*, 23(4): 44.

Institute of Medicine, Committee on Quality of Health Care in America (2001) *Crossing the Quality Chasm: A New Health System for the 21st Century*. Washington, D.C.: National Academy Press.

Johns, C. (2010) Clinical supervision: Reflective practice; learning through experience, in Cox, C. and Hill, M. (Eds), *Professional Issues in Primary Care*, Chapter 11. Oxford: Wiley-Blackwell. pp: 173–185.

Katz, J., Kessler, C., O'Connell, A. and Levine, S. (2007) Professionalism and evolving concepts of quality. *Society of General Internal Medicine*, 22(1): 137–139.

Klein, R. (2013) *The New Politics of the NHS*. (Seventh Edition), CRC Press, Taylor Francis Group, London.

Koornhof, L. (2025) Professionalism is vital. *South African Journal of Clinical Nutrition*, 38(3): i–ii. https://journals.co.za/doi/full/10.1080/16070658.2025.2555658 (accessed 7/06/2026).

Lebovits, A., Florence, I., Bathina, R. Hunko, V., Fox, M. and Bramble, C. (1997) Pain knowledge and attitudes of healthcare providers: practices characteristic differences. *The Clinical Journal of Pain*, 13(3): 237–243.

Lynch, D., Surdyk, P. and Eiser, A. (2004) Assessing professionalism: a review of literature. *Medical Teacher*, 26(4): 366–373.

Mahon, S. (2015) *Risk Assessment, Prevention and Early Detection: Seminars in Oncology Nursing*. Elsevier.

McGlynn, E. and Brook, R. (2001) Keeping quality on the policy agenda. *Health Affairs*, 20(3): 82–90.

Merriam-Webster's Collegiate Dictionary (2003) Merriam-Webster's Collegiate Dictionary, 11th Edition, Springfield Massachusetts: Merriam-Webster, Incorporated.

Merriam-Webster's Collegiate Dictionary (2022) Merriam-Webster's Collegiate Dictionary, 11th Edition, Springfield Massachusetts: Merriam-Webster, Incorporated.

NMC (2010) Consultation Document www.nmc.org.uk/globalassets/sitedocuments/standards/nmc-standards-for-pre-registration-nursing-education.pdf (Accessed 7/06/2026).

NMC (2023) Independent Report on the Regulation of Advanced Practice. (May 10, 2023). www.nuffieldtrust.org.uk/sites/default/files/2023-05/Advanced%20practice%20report%20FINAL%5B69%5D.pdf (accessed 7/06/2026).

NMC (2024) The Code. (January 4, 2024). www.nmc.org.uk/standards/code/ (Accessed 7/06/2026).

NMC (2025a) Principles of Advanced Practice. https://www.nmc.org.uk/standards/guidance/advanced-practice-principles/ (Accessed 7/06/2026).

NMC (2025b) Advanced Practice Principles for UK Nursing and Midwifery. www.nmc/org.u www.nmc.org.uk/standards/guidance/advanced-practice-principles/ (Accessed 7/06/2026).

Palmer, R., Smith, B., Kite, J. and Phongsavan, P. (2024) The socio-ecological derterminants of help-seeking practices and healthcare access among young men: a systematic review. *Health Promotion International*, 39(2):daae024. doi"10.1093/heapro/daae024. https://academic.oup.com/heapro/article/39/2/daae024/7633122 (Accessed 07/06/26).

Parastesh, S., Hosseini, M., Mohannad-Shahbolaghi, F., Maddah, S. and Ebadi, A. (2025) Exploring the new characteristics of professionalism in nursing from the perspective of experts: a qualitative Study. *Journal of Taibh University School of Medical Sciences*, Elsevier (October 7, 2025).

Plochg, T., Klazinga, N. and Starfield, B. (2009) Transforming medical professionalism to fit changing health needs. *BMC Medicine*, 7(64): 1–7.

Ruth, B., Sisco, S., Wyatt, J., Bachman, S. and Piper, T. (2008) Public health and social work: training dual professionals for the contemporary workplace. *Public Health Reports*, 2(123): 71–77.

Sherwood, G. (2024) Reflective practice and knowledge development. *International Journal of Nursing Sciences*, 11(4): 399–404. doi: 10.1016/j.ijnss.2024.08.002 (accessed 1/12/2025).

Shirjag, A., Doshmangir, L., Bayzar, M., Sergeevich Gordev, V. (2025) Primary healthcare reforms: a scoping review. *NIH, Primary Health Care Research & Development*, 26: e74. doi: 10.1017/S1463423625000271 (accessed 1/11/2026).

Shohani, M. and Zamanzadeh, V. (2017) Nurses' attitude towards professionalization and factors influencing it. *Journal of Caring Sciences*, 6(4): 345–357. doi: 10.15171/jcs.2017.033 (accessed 1/8/2026).

Sullivan, W. (1999) What is left of professionalism after managed care? *Hastings Centre Report*, 29(2): 7–13.

Tan, S.H.E. and Chin, G.F. (2023) Generational effect on nurses' work values, engagement, and satisfaction in an acute hospital. *BMC Nursing*, 22(1): 88, 10.1186/s12912-023-01256-2.

Taylor, D. (1996) Quality and professionalism in health care: a review of current initiatives in the NHS. *BMJ*, 312(7031): 626–629.

Van Herk, R., Klazinga, N. and Schepers, R. (2001) Medical audit: threat or opportunity for the medical profession. A comprehensive study of medical audit among medical specialists in general hospitals in the Netherlands and England, 1970 – 1999.

Welbourn, D. and Theodore, C. (2010) Revalidation – demonstrating continuing fitness to practice. Final Report to the Nursing and Midwifery Council, 29 June 2010. London: Matrix Knowledge Ltd.

Wood, N. (2025) A Clear Understanding of Professionalism and Its Importance. www.effy.ai/blog/professionalism-definition (accessed 1/9/2026).

CHAPTER 9

Clinical effectiveness

Nicola Whiteing

Introduction

There is a significant and growing global need for advanced practitioners to address healthcare workforce shortages, improve access to care and manage complex patient needs in an ageing population. The International Council of Nurses (ICN) report that many countries are implementing advanced practice roles in nursing in recognition of the broader responsibilities held by nurses including population health, planetary health and health system design (White et al. 2025). The roles, titles, regulatory frameworks and education for advanced practice roles vary by country. As workforce planning teams implement advanced practitioner roles it is imperative both to patients and the organisation that outcomes of care are obtained and evaluated in measuring and ensuring clinical effectiveness.

Whilst clinical effectiveness is an area that has important implications for patient outcomes, it is also a driver of individual professional growth and capability of advanced practitioners (Ominyi et al. 2025; Rothwell et al. 2021). As such, this chapter will explore ways in which outcomes related to clinical effectiveness can be obtained, implemented and evaluated for both the effectiveness of care delivery and the role of the advanced practitioner. Key areas including evidence-based practice (EBP), audit, research, patient satisfaction, the case manager role and continuing professional development will be explored.

Learning outcomes

At the conclusion of this chapter, you will be able to:

- Articulate the importance of clinical effectiveness and its key elements
- Discuss ways in which the advanced practitioner can become involved in the implementation of EBP
- Discuss the role of the advanced practitioner as a case manager drawing on relevant capabilities of practice

DOI: 10.4324/9781003609049-13

- Demonstrate awareness of tools for collecting evaluative data to review practice, noting their strengths and limitations
- Articulate ways in which the advanced practitioner can address continuing professional development activities for the benefit of the organisation and self

Background

Clinical effectiveness, together with patient safety and experience, is central to high-quality healthcare (Oben, 2020; Bastemeijer et al. 2019). It may be understood as delivering the right care, in the right way, at the right time and place, and achieving the right outcomes (ACSQHC, 2023). Clinical effectiveness is defined as the application of the best available knowledge – derived from research, clinical expertise and patient preferences – to optimise care processes and outcomes. It operates within a framework of informing, changing and monitoring practice (NHS Executive, 1996)

Key components include gathering evidence, incorporating patient perspectives where appropriate, implementing EBP, evaluating the impact of practice change and pursuing continuous improvement.

Healthcare must be driven by a cycle of continuous quality improvement that strengthens structures and processes of care, enhances patient wellbeing and reduces mortality (Endalamaw et al. 2024). Clinical effectiveness underpins this process and provides the evidence-based foundation for clinical governance (ACSQHC, 2017). Clinical governance provides the framework through which organisations and staff are held accountable for continuously improving service quality and the environments in which care is delivered. While the pillars of clinical governance vary in nomenclature across countries, common themes include clinical performance and effectiveness, risk management, education and training, patient safety, quality systems with public involvement, leadership and information management. EBP is concerned with using the best available evidence, combined with clinical expertise, to guide and improve care delivery (Ominyi et al. 2025) and is a key component of clinical governance. Advanced practitioners should ensure their contribution to clinical governance reports and the compilation of the services clinical governance portfolio by outlining existing achievements in addition to short-, medium- and long-term planned goals for the advanced practice service.

There is mounting pressure being exerted to ensure that healthcare delivery is evidence-based and clinically effective. EBP and decision making are the cornerstone of clinical effectiveness and have been consistently linked to improved quality care, patient safety, innovation and professional growth (Connor et al. 2022; Lehane et al. 2021; Ominyi et al. 2025). By integrating clinical expertise with high-quality research evidence, the advanced practitioner reduces uncertainty and gains confidence that their clinical, managerial and educational interventions are guided by a current and appropriate knowledge base (Mohamed et al. 2024). The use of research in practice is not a new concept; however, there is now greater emphasis on systematically analysing evidence, integrating it into clinical decision making and assessing its effects on patient outcomes. The concept of EBP has been driven though several government and professional documents globally, which aim for health services in which clinical, managerial and policy decisions are no longer based on tradition or ritual but on sound and pertinent information. As EBP is a priority in healthcare, advanced practitioners must develop the necessary skills to search for evidence effectively and integrate it into patient care (Lehane et al. 2021). This will enable practice to become more appropriate, timely and acceptable to the patient, the wider interprofessional team and the organisation. The advanced practitioner is in an ideal position to lead the development and implementation of EBP through actively participating in the design, implementation and evaluation of changes made to healthcare systems. Advanced practitioners have an ethical responsibility to provide and promote an evidence-based approach to enhance the quality of patient care (Connor et al. 2022). Table 9.1 (Whiteing, 2008) illustrates several ways in which the advanced practitioner can begin to get involved in the implementation of EBP and assist others in doing so.

Current practice often diverges from best practice, and implementing change presents significant challenges. While practitioners are expected to deliver EBP, many lack an understanding of the factors influencing implementation. Consequently, the adoption of EBP remains inconsistent, hindered by gaps in knowledge and organisational support (Rycroft-Malone et al. 2024). Advanced practitioners cannot implement change in isolation; they must collaborate with the interprofessional team to secure the necessary support and resources. Many practices persist due to tradition or personal preference, and although these should be aligned with EBP, not all can be addressed simultaneously. Advanced practitioners should therefore prioritise areas of practice in consultation with colleagues, ensuring alignment with the organisation's EBP, research and audit strategy to follow correct procedures and avoid duplication.

Achieving a change in practice often requires an initial shift in organisational culture or leadership (Mannion & Davies, 2018). The context in which the change occurs is frequently a key determinant of its success. As leaders in patient care, advanced practitioners must inspire staff through a shared vision rather than rely on command-and-control approaches. By adopting a transformational leadership style, advanced practitioners can foster a culture that supports the integration of evidence into practice.

EBP and the use of Integrated Care Pathways (ICPs) (refer to the following pages) have been criticised for being overly 'prescriptive' and limiting flexibility in

Table 9.1 Ways in Which the Advanced Practitioner Can Get Involved in EBP and Help Others to Be Involved

- Attendance and contribution at:
  - o Interprofessional/staff meetings
  - o Clinical governance forums
  - o Clinical practice committees
  - o Research and audit committees/meetings
- Project management
- Clinical supervision
- Provide educational opportunities and resources
- Peer mentorship
- Collaboration with higher education institutions
- Engage in scholarly inquiry
- Dissemination of findings
- Foster a supportive environment
- Expert role modelling

Adapted from Whiteing (2008).

individualised care. While this may be true for less experienced practitioners seeking guidance on patient management, advanced practitioners can use ICPs to reflect on care delivery and identify alternative approaches for individual patients or patient groups. Community matrons in the UK and Nurse Practitioners in Australia and the United States are well positioned to evaluate patient's self-management of their conditions and incorporate these insights into future care planning. A central aspect of their role is the ability to adapt care packages and pathways to accommodate individual needs and preferences. Advanced practitioners must collaborate with patients to ensure their needs are recognised and documented within ICPs, while also guiding staff to use pathways as flexible frameworks rather than rigid protocols, applying clinical judgement when planning care.

The clinically effective advanced practitioner

The advanced practitioner working as a case manager is a role that has been supported globally throughout the literature in providing effective care (Feyereisen & Puro, 2023; Htay & Whitehead, 2021). Indeed, many roles within the UK, Australia and the US have adopted the role of case manager as a means of delivering high-quality, outcome-focused care. The care needs of patients are becoming more complex with an ageing population. The case management role enables the advanced practitioner to respond proactively to the challenges inherent in coordinating complex care.

The Department of Health, in 2004, outlined the role of the community matron in which an advanced nurse practitioner provides case management for people with severe, long-term and complex health needs. Through this case management approach systematic proactive care is delivered to prevent unplanned hospital admissions and premature admission to long-term care facilities and to expedite discharge (Tregenza, 2019; DoH, 2004).

Whilst the DoH documents (2004, 2005, 2006) focus on the role of the community matron as a case manager, the content and frameworks can be applied to a range of patients being managed by the advanced practitioner in both acute and primary care environments.

Case management provides a structured approach to enhancing the coordination of healthcare services and improving access to care across populations (Joo & Liu, 2017; Putra & Sandhi, 2021). This model optimises the use of resources, strengthens communication between healthcare professionals, patients and families and supports advocacy within the healthcare system (Bashkin et al. 2023; Fabbri et al. 2017; van Voorst & Arnold, 2020). Within this framework, the advanced practitioner guides the patient's journey from assessment through to discharge or referral. Their role requires competence in obtaining medical histories, conducting physical examinations, initiating and interpreting diagnostic tests and applying critical reasoning for diagnosis and decision making. The advanced practitioner, as case manager, is also responsible for arranging consultations with specialists or specialist services and facilitating transfers to more appropriate levels of care when necessary. Regardless of the patient's care setting, they retain accountability for scheduling and reviewing test results, procedures and treatments, as well as negotiating access to primary and secondary care resources and monitoring outcomes. Collectively these responsibilities align with the core capabilities of advanced practice across the four pillars of advanced practice (NHS England, 2025a).

It is more than just the patient's presenting complaint that needs to be managed by the advanced practitioner. The advanced nurse practitioner should have an appreciation of the need for prevention or treatment of health issues (Doody et al. 2025; Tregenza, 2019). This is particularly relevant in the UK at the present time. The Comprehensive Model for Personalised Care introduced within the National Health Service (NHS) Long Term Plan represents a strategic shift towards tailoring healthcare to individual needs, preferences and circumstances (NHS England, 2019a). It emphasises shared decision making, supported self-management, personalised care planning and access to social prescribing and community-based support. By placing patients at the centre of their care, the model aims to improve health outcomes, enhance patient experience and reduce health inequalities (NHS England, 2019b). It also reflects a broader commitment within the NHS to integrate health and social care, ensuing that services are proactive, coordinated and responsive to the diverse needs of the population.

For the advanced practitioner, fulfilling the commitment to personalised care requires an emphasis on longitudinal, relationship-based case management. Recent research by Runnels et al. (2025) highlights the value of sustained relationship building between advanced practitioners and patients, demonstrating how this approach shifts away from transactional interactions towards partnership and customisation of care, leading to cost saving and enhanced quality of life.

Advanced practice offers practitioners the opportunity to redefine the traditional professional boundaries, enabling continuity and co-ordination of care through collaboration with interprofessional teams. Evidence demonstrates that interprofessional collaboration enhances person-centred care and leads to improved outcomes for patients, the workforce,and health systems (Ford et al. 2023; Squires et al. 2021; WHO 2010). Advanced practitioners, regardless of discipline, frequently provide a significant proportion of patient care activities. Within this context, it is essential that they engage with other members of the interprofessional team, collaborate in setting goals of care and draw on critical thinking, current research and diagnostic reasoning to deliver high-quality care while ensuring the efficient use of resources (Cox, 2019). Such collaboration helps to eliminate the fragmented, siloed care that often occurs as patients move between departments and professionals. Given the increasing complexity of patient needs, advanced practitioners must also be able to lead interprofessional teams when appropriate, demonstrating effective communication and collaboration across disciplines (McLaney et al. 2022).

Following patient assessment and the formulation of differential diagnoses, a care plan should be developed collaboratively with the interprofessional team. While joint goal setting is essential, advanced practitioners must recognise when patient management extends beyond their scope of practice and make appropriate referrals. In such cases, support should be sought from more experienced colleagues. Building effective relationships with other healthcare professionals is therefore critical to achieving coordinated and comprehensive patient care. The ICP, discussed later in this chapter, provides a valuable framework for enhancing communication and collaboration across professional boundaries.

Beyond the advanced practitioner's own organisation, collaboration across acute, primary and tertiary care is essential to ensure seamless transitions during referral or discharge. Engagement with the wider health and social care network is also necessary to appreciate broader issues. By developing an awareness of the roles of other healthcare professionals and the functions of different care settings, advanced practitioners are better positioned to make appropriate referrals and to identify and address variations in health, thereby contributing to improved outcomes (Goldsberry, 2018).

Evaluating responses to healthcare and revising practice

There is a continual pressure on healthcare providers to improve the quality of care, effectiveness and efficiency with which it is delivered. These are essential components to improving the patient's experience. In examining the quality-of-care delivery; the patient's response to the healthcare provided, the provider and its effectiveness must be evaluated. The advanced practitioner has several sources in which valuable data can be captured including patient records, policies, protocols, pathways, guidelines and standards, which may provide information on the patient's responses to healthcare that is planned, has been or is being delivered and its effectiveness. The advanced practitioner should identify from patients' care plans any variances from planned pathways and work with the interprofessional team, including the patient, to analyse and resolve them where possible. The following section discusses a variety of ways in which patients and organisational responses to healthcare delivery can be evaluated.

Integrated care pathways (ICPs)

ICPs are used extensively in managing patient outcomes and care processes in primary and secondary care. ICPs are complex multi-disciplinary care plans which outline a course of events for the treatment of patients with the same/similar conditions or undergoing similar procedures. This maintains standardised levels of care across settings while still ensuring care remains personalised to meet the individual needs of each patient (Jerjes & Harding, 2024). Activities are placed on a timeline which depending on the place of use and condition for which the ICP has been written will vary between hourly (e.g., in an Intensive Care Unit), daily (e.g., post-operatively on a ward) or weekly (e.g., mental health setting). All activities relating to the patient journey from initial diagnosis to long-term follow up are included, no matter which professional carries them out. Thus, the ICP enables one evidence-based tool to be used by all professionals providing care for the patient. This facilitates enhanced communication between professionals and enables team members to view patient progress in other areas that may impact on their own activities with the patient. Importantly the ICP also enables the patient to work in partnership with professionals through visible goals and activities (Grocott, 2019). This collaborative working reduces complications, ensures patient safety and supports resource utilisation through a reduced length of stay (McLaney et al. 2022; Squires et al. 2021).

The ICP is a dynamic document that should be regularly updated to reflect organisational changes and emerging research. Advanced Practitioners have a role in monitoring patient outcomes through variance tracking, which records deviations from the planned care pathway. Variances may arise when patients fail to meet expected milestones (e.g., due to physiological issues), when practitioners delay or omit treatments or when systemic factors such as limited resources or unclear policies intervene. Each variance should be documented with its cause and corrective actions. Monitoring variance frequency and causes allows trends to be identified, and practices adjusted, ensuring the pathway remains clinically effective. Advanced practitioners are well placed to become actively involved in the development and continual refinement of ICPs including engaging patients as co-designers of the care pathway (Jerjes & Harding, 2024).

Case study

A health service identified delays and inconsistent care for stroke patients, including slow diagnosis, variable rehabilitation planning, and poor coordination between hospital and community services.

An integrated care pathway (ICP) was introduced to streamline care. Key elements included early involvement of the multidisciplinary team, referral to community rehabilitation prior to discharge, and structured GP follow-up within specified timeframes.

The ICP delivered a seamless, evidence-based approach across acute, rehabilitation and community care. By reducing variation and improving communication, it enhanced both outcomes and service efficiency.

Clinical audit

The importance of clinicians carrying out audits has long been recognised as an essential activity in ensuring quality care and a core component of clinical governance. Clinical audit, unlike a survey which describes an issue, examines an activity or practice against an established or desired standard of practice (Skull, 2020). A considerable amount of single-discipline audit has been carried out over the years; however, if benefits to patients are to occur, all members of the interprofessional team need to be involved in improving care. The ICP discussed above provides a good platform for establishing such interprofessional audits. It is through regular audit and evaluation of practice that areas where services are not meeting explicit standards are identified for improvement (Foy et al. 2020) and clinically effective care is highlighted. For audit to be successful and have an impact it needs to be regarded as a continuous cycle rather than being a one-off measurement. Audit is often referred to as a cycle or a spiral to emphasise its ongoing process.

Evaluating the patient's response to healthcare and its delivery

Funding for hospitals is, in part, based on a range of quality measures such as patient safety, patient experience and effectiveness of care measured through key clinical indicators (e.g., infection rates). While several clinical measurement tools are available for measuring clinical effectiveness such as length of stay, mortality and morbidity, readmission rates, infection rates; the information gleaned from them does not give any indication as to the patient's experience of their healthcare provision nor does it demonstrate whether the patient's own desired outcomes have been met. In order that healthcare can be understood and improved it is essential that the patient's perspective is sought (Jamieson Gilmore et al. 2023; Wolf et al. 2021). It is through the use of patient-reported outcome measures (PROMs) and patient-reported experience measures (PREMs) that this data can be generated.

Patient-reported outcome measures (PROMs) and patient-reported experience measures (PREMs)

PROMs aim to capture and measure the patient's perspective of health status or health-related quality of life in a reliable, valid, acceptable and feasible way at a single point in time. The use of PROMs has been shown to improve survival, symptom control and detection of unrecognised problems, decrease readmissions and improve communication between patients and healthcare professionals (Amat-Fernandez et al. 2025). PREMs provide insight into the individual's experience and satisfaction with health service engagement (Jamieson Gilmore et al. 2023). Both are self-reported measures completed by the care recipient (Casaca et al. 2023). Quality in the context of healthcare is more than patient satisfaction and whilst patient satisfaction, as an experience, is important to measure, this alone may not ensure an impact on patient outcome, i.e., an improvement in health. Nevertheless, the use of PROMs and PREMs in combination is an effective tool for discerning high-quality care and areas for improvement. Advanced practitioners, with their clinical expertise, patient-centred focus and holistic approach to care, are well placed to gather data and implement changes to healthcare delivery after PROM/PREM data collection, assessment and evaluation (Drury et al. 2024). It is therefore vital that they understand what measures are available, how they are best utilised and importantly how the data gathered can be used to directly improve a variety of outcomes.

PROMs are usually obtained using a questionnaire although interviews can be utilised in some circumstances (Foster et al. 2018). Questionnaires used to collect PROMs can be self-, interviewer- or telephone-administered. Whichever method is used it is important that the user ensures that the tool is administered in the way for which it has been developed, or its validity will be affected. For some patients, such as those that are unable to read or write, have difficulty recalling their symptoms, are too unwell to report symptoms or have a disability affecting their ability to return a questionnaire by post, the use of a questionnaire is not the best approach to gaining information (Nguyen et al. 2021). In these circumstances a structured, semi-structured or unstructured interview or focus group can be used.

PROMs tools can be *generic* or *disease specific*. Generic tools such as the Quality of Life (EQ-5D-5L) measure (https://euroqol.org/information-and-support/euroqol-instruments/eq-5d-5l/) are widely applicable to patient populations and patient perceptions of their general 'generic' health status. Generic tools have the advantage of being suitable across a wide range of health problems and conditions; however, this does mean that the data are not generalisable to a specific population as specific data for a disease or condition is not obtained. Disease-specific tools allow data to be gathered on a particular health problem or population including disease/condition-specific tools, population-specific tools and dimension-specific tools which focus on a particular aspect of health status (Whittal et al. 2021). There are many specific tools that the advanced practitioner should familiarise themselves with to enable them to choose the most appropriate tool for the proposed application.

Several barriers have been identified to the implementation of PROMs and PREMs. These barriers can be grouped as occurring at the patient level and the health provider level (Glenwright et al. 2023; Nguyen et al. 2021; Foster et al. 2018). Patient-level barriers include the time to complete PROMs, inconvenience, unknown value of the data, unrelated responses and difficulty in using technology (Glenwright et al. 2023; Nguyen et al. 2021; Foster et al. 2018). At the health provider level, staff workload, technical difficulties, difficulty in analysing data, perceived lack of value by staff, lack of resources and staff training and a lack of tools have all been identified (Nguyen et al. 2021). Despite these barriers the general evidence on PROMs is positive and their use is encouraged globally (Amat-Fernandez et al. 2025). In the UK all NHS-funded care providers since 2009 have collected PROMs for hip and knee replacements (NHS England, 2019b). In Australia the Australian Commission on Safety and Quality in Health Care (ACSQHC) is working to support the use of PROMs to drive quality improvement through enabling the patient voice (ACSQHC, 2025a). The use of PROMs and PREMs demonstrates the advanced practitioner's contribution to the Nursing and Midwifery Council's Principles for Advanced Practice (NMC, 2025) and Pillar 1 and Pillar 2 of the Multiprofessional framework for advanced practice in England (NHS England, 2025a).

Activity 1

Consider how you could implement the use of PROMs within your patient/client group. Undertake a search for available validated tools that may be of use in gathering data in your chosen area and consider how they may inform your work as an advanced practitioner in the service you provide. Reflect on this with a colleague.

Evaluating the advanced practitioner service

In considering and ensuring clinical effectiveness, the advanced practitioner has a role not only in evaluating and improving the quality of healthcare but also in evaluating their own practice and role within the organisation. For advanced practitioners to be valued by colleagues, the organisation and the public, it is essential that their work is clearly connected to patient outcomes. Advanced practice roles are multifaceted, evolving and increasing in number (Unsworth et al. 2024; NHS England, 2023a); however, such roles need to demonstrate that they contribute to improved outcomes as reflected in the four pillars for advanced practice (NHS England, 2025a) Thus the advanced practitioner must be able to justify not only patient outcomes, but also the effectiveness of their role and service for key stakeholders such as employers, professional bodies and education providers (Scott, 2024).

There are a number of ways in which the advanced practitioner and the wider team can evaluate the impact of advanced practice services including: audit, research, patient satisfaction surveys and feedback to the individual practitioner or team.

Audit trails

The role of clinical audit has been discussed previously in its contribution to ensuring clinical effectiveness. Alongside clinical audits an outcomes audit of those patients managed by the advanced practitioner will help inform policy makers and organisations in their decision making regarding the advanced practitioner role and how it can be best used to enhance patient care (Thompson et al. 2025). Simple records of activity, referrals, trends and clinical outcomes can provide the advanced practitioner and the organisation with valuable data which should be used to produce activity and outcome reports to service managers as applicable. In monitoring the effectiveness and quality of the advanced practitioner service the patient's progress should be tracked once they have left their care. This may be difficult for some advanced practitioners to do, particularly those working in areas such as urgent care centres, emergency departments and minor injury units. For the advanced practitioner working in a General Practice (GP) surgery, however, it is much easier to follow the patient up with a phone call to ensure that they are progressing well and to monitor such factors as complication rates, readmission to services and satisfaction with services.

Peer audit as part of a broader peer review also offers the opportunity to formally or informally examine the quality of the advanced practice role or service against a set of professional standards (Fedel et al. 2019). A group of people of equal qualification/grade assess the performance of the advanced practitioner. Achieving successful audit of any type is not without difficulties and as such the advanced practitioner needs to ensure familiarity with the organisation's audit strategy, a model for use and an environment that recognises the value of audit in ensuring clinical effectiveness.

Research

Research is fundamental to enhancing both patient outcomes and the overall quality of healthcare (Janerka et al. 2024). Healthcare professions globally have made considerable advances in becoming research-driven professions with several national strategies supporting the healthcare workforce to ensure research capacity is built and evidence is embedded into practice and professional decision making (NHS England, 2021a, 2025b; NHS Health Education England, 2022; NHS England, 2023b; Department of Health and Aged Care, 2024).

Advanced Practitioners are well placed to contribute to, and lead research, and this is recognised in the NHS England Multi-professional framework for advanced practice (NHS England, 2025a, 2025b), where research capabilities are defined in the fourth pillar of advanced practice (research). While recognising that research, along with the other three pillars, will form the basis of an advanced practice role, what this looks like for each individual practitioner will differ dependent on their prior skills, qualifications, role, organisation and service delivery. Some practitioners will have the capabilities to support, deliver or lead research while others may not yet be best positioned to do so. Despite this, however, all practitioners must make considered use of research evidence to inform their decision making (NHS England, 2024). Advanced practitioners must therefore be able to critically appraise and synthesise relevant research and use the results to guide their own practice and that of others through dissemination of best practice (NHS England, 2025a).

To enable a rigorous evaluation of the advanced practitioner service, the advanced practitioner should work towards gaining an understanding of the research process and research methodologies and grow their research capacity. This will enable them to participate in or lead research into the impact of their service delivery and continuously improve and contribute to EBP as discussed at the beginning of this chapter. Challenges contributing to low levels of research activity among advanced practitioners include inadequate protected time, limited confidence and competence in research skills and application and insufficient support and resources (Casey & O'Connor, 2022; Strachan et al. 2022).

The central requirement in evaluating effectiveness is the measurement of actual practice, such as that of an advanced practitioner, against an established standard or benchmark, for example, results achieved by similar practitioners/services, internally established targets or professional standards. While research capturing a service at a particular timepoint is useful, there is a need for longitudinal research to be undertaken to examine the diverse and evolving work of advanced practitioners (Scott, 2024). Services delivered by an advanced practitioner are often compared to those of medical practitioners; however, due to the very nature of the advanced practice role, in particular the nurse as an advanced practitioner, the two services will be very different and cannot be judged by the same markers. The advanced practice nurse, perhaps more so than other health professionals working at an advanced level, will spend much longer during a consultation due to the holistic approach taken, spending extra time on health education and addressing emotional and social elements. Whilst this may have cost implications to the organisation, in relation to time spent and productivity in ensuring clinical effectiveness, from the patient's perspective this is an important and valued aspect of service delivery.

Valid research evidence is essential both to counter opposition to advanced practice services and to sustain ongoing investment in them (Alla & Joss, 2021). The research undertaken by advanced practitioners must be written up to fulfil their role in contributing to evidence-based practice and service improvement. This may take the form of a written report for the organisation; however, opportunities to disseminate work more broadly should also be undertaken. This may include writing for publication or conference presentations.

Patient satisfaction surveys

The public's expectations of their own treatment and healthcare services are increasingly used as key quality indicators (Friedel at al. 2023). Patient satisfaction surveys are commonplace and are useful in obtaining data relating to how patients have viewed the quality of a service; however, the data gathered is opinion focused and subjective (ACSQHC, 2025b). Most patient satisfaction surveys are carried out via a questionnaire which has been developed by an individual asking their chosen questions. Satisfaction surveys often give an over-optimistic view, particularly where outcomes of care (e.g., post-surgery) have been positive, thus not highlighting areas of poor care delivery. Patient satisfaction is dependent on the patient's individual level of expectations of services, and this is based on multiple factors including their culture and social circumstances (Lakin & Kane, 2022); in addition, patients often do not have clear reasons for their evaluations. For these reasons a follow up telephone conversation in which answers can be explored further may be useful in gathering data with greater meaning.

Gathering data on patient satisfaction is extremely important in ensuring the provision of clinically effective care. Other audit measures will not obtain such data. The pitfalls of the patient satisfaction survey have been highlighted, and the advanced practitioner should consider the use of PROMs and PREMs (as discussed earlier) alongside such surveys. The advantage PROMs and PREMs have over routine self-developed patient satisfaction surveys is that they have been validated for their specific use and therefore data are expected to have more validity.

Feedback

Feedback from within and external to the advanced practitioner's organisation can be helpful in developing services. This may be informal feedback through meetings or networking forums or more formal, utilising the appraisal process or 360-degree evaluation, which provides a holistic and comprehensive assessment of an individual (Cormack et al. 2018). 360-degree feedback is a process whereby the advanced practitioners' own ratings as to his/her performance are compared to those ratings given anonymously by colleagues. Advanced practitioners must continue to develop their role in response to feedback received and demonstrate its effectiveness in clinical care, providing strong leadership and communicating the role's purpose, scope and education.

> **Activity 2**
> Choose an aspect of your clinical practice; consider how you might go about obtaining evidence, implementing a change and evaluating the impact of the change in your chosen area.

Maintaining competence through continuing professional development

Advanced practitioners are personally and professionally accountable for their own practice and as such must ensure their own competence to undertake the advanced practice activities to the same standard as the professional that would have traditionally undertaken them. Clinical effectiveness becomes compromised when advanced practitioners are poorly prepared for their roles and possess insufficient knowledge and skills. All healthcare professionals working at the level of an advanced practitioner are required to consistently meet the capabilities under each of the four pillars of Advanced Practice (Lee, 2021; NHS England, 2025a). In working to these expected capabilities, advanced practitioners will need to possess and apply an extensive repertoire of skills. To continue to be able to apply such skills, the advanced practitioner primarily engages with clinical work which requires an ability to utilise evidence in their decision making to inform clinical reasoning. The need to maintain competence through continuing professional development (CPD) and lifelong learning is essential, demonstrating a commitment to excellence (Doody et al. 2025; Kurtović et al. 2024). The final part of this chapter will offer some suggestions as to ways in which the advanced practitioner can achieve this.

The importance of CPD cannot be underestimated. It is crucial for maintaining competence, patient safety and professional standards (King et al. 2021) in a rapidly evolving healthcare world (Graebe 2024; Graebe et al. 2022). There are many recognised CPD activities, some that focus on improving the healthcare environment, some that focus on self-development and others that focus on both. CPD activities can include but are not limited to conducting research, sharing of information at public forums, promotion of EBP and outcomes measurement, pursuing higher education, writing for publication, attendance at organised learning events, structured learning such as an Advanced Life Support (ALS) course, reflection, professional supervision and E-learning.

It is evident that CPD includes much more than higher education courses or simply staying current. Indeed, for CPD to be effective it is crucial that there is a relationship between CPD activities, organisational context and culture for learning to be transferred to the workplace (Jackson & Manley, 2022; Marvin et al. 2010). The advanced practitioner must ensure that initial training is consolidated through practice and that personal priorities for professional growth and career satisfaction are established and made known to employers. To support advanced practitioners in considering their CPD requirements the Centre for Advancing Practice provides guidance to professionals in how their CPD, and growth can be aligned with the four pillars of advanced practice (NHS England, 2021b).

While the extent to which a practitioner will work in each pillar will vary depending on role and experience, all four pillars must be actively engaged with. Advanced practitioners must be competent in the assessment, diagnosis, treatment and care of patients whilst forming and maintaining genuine partnerships with them. To ensure clinical credibility and impact the advanced practitioner must therefore be seen to be participating in these clinical roles (Mann et al. 2023; Htay & Whitehead, 2021) despite someone's core business being in education or leadership, for example. The advanced practitioner can attend short courses and study days, shadow other members of staff within and outside of their organisation and actively participate in specialist interest groups and professional forums.

CPD activities can develop not only the individual practitioner but also the organisation and advanced practitioners now have opportunities to obtain positions in which time may be allocated to writing, undertaking research, public speaking, teaching and consulting. In ensuring that practice stays up to date and therefore clinically effective the advanced practitioner may want to become involved in teaching outside of their organisation such as at a university, writing for publication, sitting on editorial or review boards and attending and speaking at local, national and international conferences. The multi-professional practice-based research capabilities framework (NHS England, 2024) is a useful document to guide practitioners at all levels to support, deliver or lead research. The framework can assist practitioners in identifying their own areas for development which may be met through CPD.

Professional supervision is a formal, confidential and critically reflective process where an experienced supervisor guides a less experienced professional (supervisee) to enhance their skills, knowledge, ethical practice and wellbeing. For trainee advanced practitioners in the UK, one hour of professional supervision per week is mandatory, with more than one supervisor possibly being needed to ensure all four pillars are met (NHS England, 2020). Supervision can take many different forms including critical reflection of clinical cases, action learning sets, facilitated discussions, case-based discussions and identification of development needs (Lee et al. 2022; ACMHN et al. 2019). While not mandatory, the benefits of continuing professional supervision once the health professional has transitioned into an advanced practitioner role are evident (Evans et al. 2021; Mann et al. 2023), particularly in managing the demands of practice and supporting professional wellbeing. A variety of approaches to supervision can be utilised including one-to-one supervision, group supervision and network supervision (Kingsley et al. 2023). Advanced practice roles can sometimes be isolating so the opportunity to meet with others in a professional supervision group can also be of benefit to the practitioner both in developing clinically effective practice and as a social support mechanism, decreasing emotional fatigue burnout and attrition. This is particularly so in rural and remote areas found in countries such as Australia and Northern America and in nurse-led clinics (Kingsley et al. 2023; Ryan et al, 2020).

Activity 3

Consider your own role either as an advanced practitioner already or in working towards this. How are you meeting the capabilities for advanced practice (NHS England, 2025a)? Reflect on those pillars that you may not be fully meeting. Consider whether this has an impact on organisational effectiveness and care delivery. In what ways could you improve clinical effectiveness by developing these capabilities? What are your CPD needs to help you develop in these areas?

Conclusion

Measuring clinical effectiveness should not just be about the identification of potentially poor practice or performance but should be about learning from and disseminating good practice between individuals, departments and healthcare providers both locally and nationally. This chapter has looked at clinical effectiveness and ways in which the advanced practitioner can obtain and implement evidence and evaluate the impact of changed practices. In ensuring a clinically effective service it is not enough to focus purely on organisational targets and clinical outcomes; the views of patients must also be obtained if quality healthcare is to be assured.

Those practitioners working at an advanced level hold a privileged, innovative and exciting role; one in which they have the opportunity to facilitate the patient's journey through each stage of the healthcare system, monitoring and ensuring effectiveness through a variety of means. These roles, however, may be open to criticism and it is therefore important that the advanced practitioner is able to provide evidence that organisational outcomes are being achieved and improved upon and that the needs of the patients are ultimately being met.

References

Alla, K., & Joss, N. (2021). *What is an evidence-informed approach to practice and why is it important?* Australian Institute of Family Studies. https://aifs.gov.au/resources/short-articles/what-evidence-informed-approach-practice-and-why-it-important#:~:text=The%20inclusion%20of%20research%20in,social%20and%20health%20care%20research.

Amat-Fernandez, C., Pardo, Y., Ferrer, M., Bosch, G., Lizano-Barrantes, C., Briseño-Diaz, R., Vernet-Tomas, M., … Hospital de Mar Patient-Reported Measures Group. (2025). Evaluating the implementation of PROMs and PREMs in routine clinical care: co-design of tools from the perspective of patients and healthcare professionals. *Health and Quality of Life Outcomes 23*(15). doi:10.1186/s12955-025-02333-7

Australian College of Mental Health Nurses [ACMHN], Australian College of Midwives [ACM] & Australian College of Nursing [CAN]. (2019). *Position Statement Clinical Supervision for Nurses and Midwives. chrome-extension://efaidnbmnnnibpcajpcglclefindmkaj* / www.acn.edu.au/wp-content/uploads/clinical-supervision-nurses-midwives-position-statement-background-paper.pdf

Australian Commission on Safety and Quality in Health Care [ACSQHC]. (2017). *National Model Clinical Governance Framework*. Sydney: ACSQHC.

Australian Commission on Safety and Quality in Health Care [ACSQHC]. (2023). *Delivering on 'right care, right place, right time'. How clinical care standards are improving health care in Australia: an evaluation report for the Antimicrobial Stewardship, Delirium and Hip Fracture Care Clinical Care Standards*. ACSQHC, Sydney.

Australian Commission on Safety and Quality in Health Care [ACSQHC]. (2025a). *Patient-reported outcome measures. ACSQHC.* www.safetyandquality.gov.au/our-work/indicators-measurement-and-reporting/patient-reported-outcome-measures.

Australian Commission on Safety and Quality in Health Care [ACSQHC]. (2025b). *Patient Experience.* www.safetyandquality.gov.au/our-work/indicators-measurement-and-reporting/patient-experience

Bashkin, O., Asna, N., Amoyal, M., & Dopelt, K. (2023). The role of nurses in the quality of cancer care management: Perceptions of cancer survivors and oncology teams. *Seminars in Oncology Nursing 39*. doi:10.1016/j.soncn.2023.151423.

Bastemeijer, C. M., Boosman, H., van Ewijk, H., Verweij, L. M., Voogt, L., & Hazelzet, J. A. (2019). Patient experiences: A systematic review of quality improvement interventions in a hospital setting. *Patient Related Outcome Measures 10*, 157–169. doi:10.2147/PROM.S201737.

Casaca, P., Schäfer, W., Nunes, A. B., & Sousa, P. (2023). Using patient-reported outcome measures and patient-reported experience measures to elevate the quality of healthcare. *International Journal for Quality in Health Care 35*(4), 1–2. doi:10.1093/intqhc/mzad098.

Casey, M., & O'Connor, L., (2022). Advanced practice nursing: Should research be the icing on the cake. *Nursing Open 9*(1), 8. doi:10.1002/nop2.1122.

Connor, L., Dean, J., McNett, M., Tydings, D. M., Shrout, A., Gorsuch, P. F., Hole, A., … Gallagher-Ford, L. (2022). Evidence-based practice improves patient outcomes and healthcare system return on investment: Findings from a scoping review. *Worldviews on Evidence-Based Nursing 20*, 6–15. doi:10.1111/wvn.12621.

Cormack, C. L., Jensen, E., Durham, C. O., Smith, G., & Dumas, B. (2018). The 360-degree evaluation model: A method for assessing competency in graduate nursing students. A pilot research study. *Nurse Education Today 64*, 132–137. doi:10.1016/j.nedt.2018.01.027.

Cox, C. (2019). *Physical Assessment for Nurses*. 3rd edn. Oxford: Wiley-Blackwell.

Department of Health. (2004). *NHS Improvement Plan 2004: Putting people at the heart of public services*. London: HMSO.

Department of Health. (2005). *Case management competencies framework for the care of people with long term conditions*. London: HMSO.

Department of Health. (2006). *Caring for people with long term conditions an education framework for community matrons and case managers*. London: HMSO.

Department of Health & Aged Care. (2024). *National Nursing Workforce Strategy – Volume 2: Research Report*. Australian Government. www.health.gov.au/our-work/national-nursing-workforce-strategy?language=en

Doody, O., Graham, M., Hegarty, O., Sloane, A. M., Walsh, P., Synott, M., Russell, M., … Murphy, L. (2025). Identifying the landscape and contribution of advanced nurse practitioners in supporting healthcare provision in Ireland in the 21st century: An integrative review. *International Journal of Nursing Studies Advances* 8. doi:10.1016/j.ijnsa.2025.100304.

Drury, A., Boland, V., & Dowling, M. (2024). Patient-reported outcome and experience measures in advanced nursing practice: What are key considerations for implementation and optimized use? *Seminars in Oncology Nursing 40*. doi:10.1016/j.soncn.2024.151632.

Endalamaw, A., Khatri, R. B., Mengistu, T. S., Erku, D., Wolka, E., Zewdie, A., & Assefa, Y. (2024). A scoping review of continuous quality improvement in healthcare systems: conceptualization, models and tools, barriers and facilitators, and impact. *BMC Health Services Research 12,* 487. doi:10.1186/s12913-024-10828-0.

Evans, C., Poku, B., Pearce, R., Eldridge, J., Hendrick, P., Knaggs, R., Blake, H., ...Collier, R. (2021). Characterising the outcomes, impacts and implementation challenges of advanced clinical practice roles in the UK: A scoping review. *BMJ Open 11*(8). doi:10.1136/bmjopen-2020-048171.

Fabbri, E., DeMaria, M., & Bertolaccini, L. (2017). Case management: An up to date review of literature and a proposal of a county utilization. *Annals of Translational Medicine 5*(20), 396. doi:10.21037/atm.2017.07.26.

Fedel, P. R., Hembel, N. E., & Mueller, L. M. (2019). Creation of a palliative care advanced practice registered nurse peer-review process. *International Journal of Palliative Nursing 25*(12), 596–602. doi:10.12968/ijpn.2019.25.12.596.

Feyereisen, S., & Puro, N. (2023). Advanced practice nurse case managers improve efforts by US hospitals to address patient social needs. *Journal of Advanced Nursing 80*(6), 2577–2583. doi: 10.1111/jan.15937.

Ford, M., Martin, P., & Sy, M. (2023). Twelve tips to support healthcare teams to incorporate interprofessional education and collaborative practice into day-to-day workplace practices. *Journal of Practice Teaching & Learning 19*(3), 6–23. doi:10.1921/jpts.v19i3.1835.

Foster, A., Croot, L., Brazier, J., Harris, J., & O'Cathain, A. (2018). The facilitators and barriers to implementing patient reported outcome measures in organisations delivering health related services: a systematic review of reviews. *Journal of Patient-Reported Outcomes 2*(46). doi:10.1186/s41687-018/-0072-3.

Foy, R., Skrypak, M., Alderson, S., Ivers, N. M., McInerney, B., Stoddart, J., Ingham, J., & Keenan, D. (2020). Revitalising audit and feedback to improve patient care. *BMJ* 368. doi:10.1136/bmj.m213.

Friedel, A. L., Siegel, S., Kirstein, C. F., Gerigk, M., Bingel, U., Diehl, A., Steidle, O., ... Kreitschmann-Andermahr, I. (2023). Measuring patient experience and patient satisfaction – how are we doing it and why does it matter? A comparison of European and U.S. American approaches. *Healthcare 11*(6), 797. doi:10.3390/healthcare11060797.

Glenwright, B. G., Simmich, J., Cottrell, M., O'Leary, S. P., Sullivan, C., Pole, J. D., & Russell, T. (2023). Facilitators and barriers to implementing electronic patient-reported outcome and experience measures in a health care setting: a systematic review. *Journal of Patient-Reported Outcomes 7*(13). doi: 10.1186/s41687-023-00554-2.

Goldsberry, J. W. (2018). Advanced practice nurses leading the way: Interprofessional collaboration. *Nurse Education Today 65*, 1–3. doi:10.1016/j.nedt.2018.02.024.

Graebe, J. (2024). Advancing nursing practice: The evolution and impact of continuing professional development. *The Journal of Continuing Education in Nursing 55*(4), 153–156. doi:10.3928/00220124-20240318-02

Graebe, J., McIntyre-Hite, L., & Monaghan, D. (2022). The future of workforce development in professional nursing practice. *The Journal of Continuing Education in Nursing 53*(6), 341–343. doi:10.3928/00220124-20230711-02.

Grocott, M. P. W. (2019). Pathway redesign: Putting patients ahead of professionals. *Clinical Medicine 19*(6), 468–472. doi:10.7861/clinmed.2019-0292.

Htay, M., & Whitehead, D. (2021). The effectiveness of the role of advanced nurse practitioners compared to physician-led or usual care: A systematic review. *International Journal of Nursing Studies Advances* 3. doi:10.1016/j.ijnsa.2021.100034.

Jackson, C., & Manley, K. (2022). Contemporary challenges of nursing CPD: Time to change the model to reflect citizens needs. *Nursing Open 9*, 880–891. doi:10.1002/nop2.941.

Jamieson Gilmore, K., Corazza, I., Coletta, L., & Allin, S. (2023). The uses of Patient Reported Experience Measures in health systems: A systematic narrative review. *Health Policy 128*, 1–10. doi:10.1016/j.healthpol.2022.07.008.

Janerka, C., Leslie, G. D., Gallagher, O., Mellan, M., Lane, M., & Gill, F. G. (2024). Understanding research capacity and culture of nurses and midwives in two health services in Western Australia. *Collegian 31*(3), 137–143. doi:10.1016/j.colegn.2024.02.001.

Jerjes, W., & Harding, D. (2024). Enhancing primary care through integrated care pathways: a convergence of theory and practice. *Frontiers in Health Services 4*. doi:10.3389/frhs.2024.1432901.

Joo, J. Y., & Liu, M. F. (2017). Case management effectiveness in reducing hospital use: a systematic review. *International Nursing Review 64*, 296–308. doi:10.1111/inr.12335.

King, R., Taylor, B., Talpur, A., Jackson, C., Manley, K., Ashby, N., Tod, A., … Robertson, S. (2021). Factors that optimise the impact of continuing professional development in nursing: A rapid evidence review. *Nurse Education Today 98*. doi:10.1016/j.nedt.2020.104652.

Kingsley, M., Hussain, F., & Ma, R. (2023). Level 2 CS for community practitioners working with palliative and end-of-life care patients. *British Journal of Nursing 32*(2), 66–72. doi:10.12968/bjon.2023.32.2.66

Kurtović, B., Gulić, P., Čukljek, S., Sedić, B., Smrekar, M., & Fičko, S. L. (2024). The commitment to excellence: Understanding nurses' perspectives on continuous professional development. *Healthcare 12*(3), 379. doi: 10.3390/healthcare12030379.

Lakin, K., & Kane, S. (2022). Peoples' expectations of healthcare: A conceptual review and proposed analytical framework. *Social Science & Medicine 292*. doi:10.1016/j.socscimed.2021.114636.

Lee, G. A. (2021). Don't forget the leadership in advanced practice. *Journal of Nursing Management 29*(4), 607–608. doi:10.1111/jonm.13032.

Lee, G. A., Baker, E. E., Stewart, C., & Raleigh, M. (2022). Advanced practice and clinical supervision: An exploration of perceived facilitators and barriers in practice. *Journal of Clinical Nursing 32*, 780–788. doi:10.1111/jocn.16341.

Lehane, E., Agreli, H., O'Connor, S., Hegarty, J., Leahy Warren, P., Bennett, D., Blake, C., … Savage, E. (2021). Building capacity: getting evidence-based practice into healthcare professional curricula. *BMJ Evidence-Based Medicine 26*(5), 1–7. doi:10.1136/bmjebm-2020-111385.

Mann, C., Timmons, S., Evans, C., Pearce, R., Overton, C., Hinsliff-Smith, K., & Conway, J. (2023). Exploring the role of advanced clinical practitioners (ACPs) and their contribution to health services in England: A qualitative exploratory study. *Nurse Education in Practice 67*. doi:10.1016/j.nepr.2023.103546.

Mannion, R., & Davies, H. (2018). Understanding organisational culture for healthcare quality improvement. *BMJ 363*. doi:10.1136/bmj.k4907.

Marvin, S., Lee, L., & Robson, F. (2010). *The evaluation of learning and development in the workplace: A review of literature*. Higher Education Funding Council for England.

McLaney, E., Morassaei, S., Hughes, L., Davies, R., Campbell, M., & Di Prospero, L. (2022). A framework for interprofessional team collaboration in a hospital setting: Advancing team competencies and behaviours. *Healthcare Management Forum 35*(2), 112–117. doi:10.1177/08404704211063584.

Mohamed, R. A., Alhujaily, M., Ahmed, F. A., Nouh, W. G., & Almowafy, A. A. (2024). *Nursing Open 11*(1). doi:10.1002/nop2.2080.

Nguyen, H., Butow, P., Dhillon, H., & Sundaresan, P. (2021). A review of the barriers to using Patient-Reported Outcomes (PROs) and Patient-Reported Outcome Measures (PROMs) in routine cancer care. *Journal of Medical Radiation Sciences 68*, 186–195. doi:10.1002/jmrs.421.

NHS England. (2019a). *Fit for the Future 10 Year Health Plan for England Executive Summary*. www.england.nhs.uk/long-term-plan/

NHS England. (2019b). *Universal Personalised Care Implementing the Comprehensive Model*. NHS England. www.england.nhs.uk/personalisedcare/comprehensive-model/

NHS England. (2020). *Minimum Standards for Supervision*. NHS England. https://advanced-practice.hee.nhs.uk/our-work/supervision/minimum-standards-for-supervision/

NHS England. (2021a). *Making Research Matter: Chief Nursing Officer for England's Strategic Plan (Version 2)*. NHS England. B0880-cno-for-englands-strategic-plan-fo-research.pdf

NHS England. (2021b). *Signpost for Continuing Professional Development*. NHS England. https://advanced-practice.hee.nhs.uk/signpost-for-continuing-professional-development/

NHS England. (2023a). *NHS Long Term Workforce Plan*. NHS England. https://www.england.nhs.uk/publication/nhs-long-term-workforce-plan/.

NHS England. (2023b). *Chief Midwifery Officer for England's Strategic Plan for Research. NHS England*. NHS England » Chief Midwifery Officer for England's Strategic Plan for Research.

NHS England. (2024). *Multi-Professional Practice-Based Research Capabilities Framework*. NHS England. https://advanced-practice.hee.nhs.uk/our-work/research/multi-professional-practice-based-research-capabilities-framework/

NHS England. (2025a). *Multi-Professional Framework for Advanced Practice in England*. NHS England. https://advanced-practice.hee.nhs.uk/multi-professional-framework-for-advanced-practice/

NHS England. (2025b). *Patient Reported Outcome Measures (PROMs)*. NHS England. www.england.nhs.uk/statistics/statistical-work-areas/proms/

NHS Executive. (1996). *Promoting Clinical Effectiveness: A Framework for Action in and Through the NHS*. Leeds: Department of Health.

NHS Health Education England. (2022). *Allied Health Professions' Research and Innovation Strategy for England*. NHS England. HEE Allied Health Professions Research and Innovation Strategy.

Nursing & Midwifery Council [NMC]. (2025). *Principles for Advanced Practice*. chrome-extension://efaidnbmnnnibpcajpcglclefindmkaj/https://www.nmc.org.uk/globalassets/sitedocuments/advanced-practice-review/principles-for-advanced-practice-english.pdf.

Oben, P. (2020). Understanding the patient experience: A conceptual framework. *Journal of Patient Experience* 7(6), 906–910. doi:10.1177/2374373520951672.

Ominyi, J., Nwedu, A., Agom, D., & Eze, U. (2025). Leading evidence-based practice: Nurse managers' strategies for knowledge utilisation in acute care settings. *BMC Nursing 24*, 252. doi:10.1186/s12912-025-02912-5.

Putra, A. D. M., & Sandhi, A., (2021). Implementation of nursing case management to improve community access to care: A scoping review. *Belitung Nursing Journal* 7(3), 141–150. doi:10.33546/bnj.1449.

Rothwell, C., Kehoe, A., Farhene Farook, S., & llling, J. (2021). Enablers and barriers to effective clinical supervision in the workplace: A rapid evidence review. *BMJ Open* 11 (9). doi:10.1136/bmjopen-2021-052929.

Runnels, P., Muskin, R., Votruba, M., Pronovost, P. J., Ansah, A., & Penman, J. (2025). Longitudinal, relationship-based case management: A prospective cohort trial. The *American Journal of Managed Care 31*(5), 216–221. doi:10.37765/ajmc.2025.89731.

Ryan, C., Cant, R., Hughes, L., Luders, E., Cooper, S., Ossenberg, C., Ahchay, D., & Fitzgerald, M. (2020). Upskilling Australian registered nurses to enhance students' clinical placement experiences: A contemporary discussion. *Australian Journal of Advanced Nursing 39*(3), 54–59. doi:10.37464/2020.393.645

Rycroft-Malone, J., Seers, K., Crichton, N., et al. (2024). Sustaining EBP through leadership and mentorship. *Journal of Nursing Management 32*(2), 240–251.

Scott, V. (2024). Assessing the benefits of advanced clinical practice for key stakeholders. *British Journal of Nursing 33*(6), 300–305. doi:10.12968/bjon.2024.33.6.300.

Skull, S. (2020). Embedding clinical audit into everyday practice: Essential methodology for all clinicians. *Journal of Paediatrics and Child Health 56*(10), 1533–1536. doi:10.1111/jpc.15068.

Squires, A., Miner, S., Greenberg, S. A., Adams, J., Kalet, A., & Cortes, T. (2021). Graduate level health professions education: how do previous work experiences influence perspectives about interprofessional collaboration? *Journal of Interprofessional Care 35*(2), 193–199.

Strachan, H., Hoskins, G., Wells, M., & Maxwell, M. (2022). A realist evaluation case study of the implementation of advanced nurse practitioner roles in primary care in Scotland. *Journal of Advanced Nursing 78*(9), 2916–2932. doi:10.1111/jan.15252.

Thompson, J., Crellin, D., Kinney, S., Matthews, S., & Gerdtz, M. (2025). Metrics used by nurse practitioners to evaluate the impact of their role: A scoping review. Science Direct, *32*(4), 183–194.

Tregenza, L. (2019). The role of the community matron: A structured approach to case management. *Nursing Older People 31*(6), 28–32. doi:10.7748/nop.2019.e1151.

Unsworth, J., Greene, K., Ali, P., Lillebo, G., & Mazilu, D. C. (2024). Advanced practice nursing roles in Europe: Implementation challenges, progress and lessons learnt. *International Nursing Review 71*(2), 299–308. doi:10.1111/inr.12800.

Van Voorst, H., & Arnold, A. E. R. (2020). Cost and health effects of case management compared with outpatient clinic follow-up in a Dutch heart failure cohort. *ESC Heart Failure 7*(3), 1136–1144. doi:10.1002/ehf2.12692.

White, J., Gunn, M., Chiarella, M., Catton, H., & Stewart, D. (2025). *Renewing the definitions of 'nursing' and 'a nurse'*. Final project report, June 2025. International Council of Nurses.

Whiteing, N. L. (2008). Domain 7: Monitoring and ensuring the quality of health care practice. In: Hinchliff, S. and Rogers, R. (Eds.), *Competencies for Advanced Nursing Practice*. London: Hodder Arnold. pp. 192–219.

Whittal, A., Meregaglia, M., & Nicod, E. (2021). The use of patient-reported outcome measures in rare diseases and implications for health technology assessment. *The Patient-Patient-Centered Outcomes Research 14*(5), 485–503. doi:10.1007/s40271-020-00493-w.

Wolf, J. A., Niederhauser, V., Marshburn, D., & LaVela, S. L. (2021). Re-examining defining patient experience: The human experience in healthcare. *Patient Experience Journal 8*(1), 16–29. doi:10.35680/2372-0247.1594.

World Health Organisation [WHO]. (2010). *Framework for Action on Interprofessional Education & Collaborative Practice*. WHO: Switzerland. www.who.int/publications/i/item/framework-for-action-on-interprofessional-education-collaborative-practice

CHAPTER 10

Influencing others

Insights from coaching and coaching psychology

Kathryn Waddington

Introduction

This chapter has been extensively revised and updated for the second edition of the book to bring a more explicit emphasis on coaching and coaching psychology theory, methods and skills. Whilst the chapter previously included reference to coaching and coaching resources, the rationale for bringing these into the foreground here is twofold. Firstly, since writing for the first edition I have retired from academic life in healthcare and psychology and I now practise and publish as a chartered coaching psychologist. Secondly, coaching is now seen as essential to supporting leadership and advanced practice development in healthcare professions (Hunaiti, 2024). For example, an executive nurse director in Kelly et al.'s (2023) qualitative study into the factors that strengthen and support more effective nurse leadership stated:

> I have a coach, I would not be able to do this job without a coach because they are the only true independent source that you have, it's a lonely job, everybody has an agenda and therefore, the only true person that you have to assist you is *yourself* and an *objective coach* [emphasis added] and that sounds quite difficult doesn't it, and it is at times.
>
> (p. 3814)

The chapter argues that ability to influence others is at the heart of leadership; and that coaching and coaching psychology are central to leadership development in turbulent times. The chapter is written in a deliberately different, creative and personalised way. Writing that is personal reveals the imperfections and weaknesses that we have traditionally been taught to hide behind 'a disembodied mask of depersonalised academic professionalism' (Boncori, 2022, p. 21). The chapter includes insights from systems-psychodynamic thinking (Sher & Lawler, 2022), which I use as a theoretical foundation in my practice as a coaching psychologist. Systems-psychodynamic thinking 'lifts the lid' on organisational life, finding the flaws and fractures found there and looking at them

DOI: 10.4324/9781003609049-14

with fresh eyes. This helps us see, hear and better understand what lies beneath the surface to gain a better understanding of – and new ways of thinking about – power and vulnerability. I am mindful that this approach and personalised way of writing may be unfamiliar to readers, who may need patience and imagination on their coaching journey with me in this chapter. It should not be read in the traditional way that professionals and academics normally read – by distilling facts, key words and references, focussing on introduction and conclusions and filtering out what we might unconsciously consider as background noise. I hope there is no unnecessary noise in this chapter; but if I succeed in my intention to write differently, readers will need to read differently.

Therefore I invite you to approach this chapter 'as if' you are engaging in a critically reflective dialogue with me, and the materials and resources here that you are reading and thinking with. This reflects a co-creative coaching partnership approach which goes beyond limited (and limiting) performance-orientated and goal-driven agendas of everyday practice in healthcare. Janelle Adsit's (2025) book *Writing and Health Care: Creative and Critical Approaches* illustrates how creative approaches resist the limitations of linear thinking and can contribute to the transformation of health systems and processes. Critical reflection involves noticing and challenging power hierarchies, assumptions and values. Research into critical reflection demonstrates its role in making healthcare more collaborative and equitable, and Edelist et al. (2024, p. 1166, emphasis in original) argue that 'dialogue as and for critical reflection should be explicitly developed within team-based healthcare.' Figure 10.1 is a framework I use in my own coaching practice – you may have other preferred frameworks/approaches that work for you.

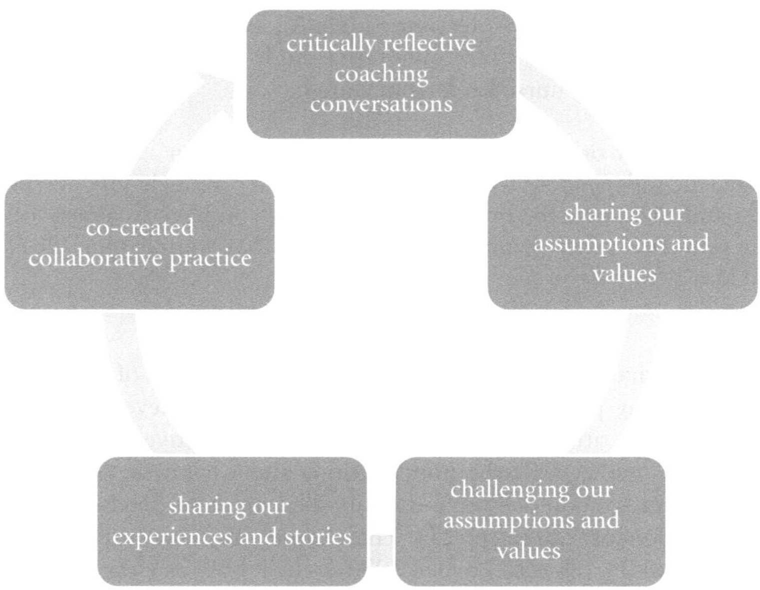
critically reflective
coaching
conversations
sharing our
assumptions and
values
challenging our
assumptions and
values
sharing our
experiences and stories
co-created
collaborative practice

Figure 10.1 Framework for critical reflection
Source: Adapted from Waddington and Jones (2023, p. 96).

Creativity, critical reflection and reflexivity are core themes that run throughout this chapter. In a world of constant change leadership and leadership development are an ongoing process. Reflexivity in the practice of leadership complements and strengthens critical reflection in the way that it helps to find 'strategies to question our own attitudes, thought processes, values, assumptions, prejudices and habitual actions' (Robson, 2022, p. xix). The traditional approach to reflection can be rather passive, while the best reflexive practice happens when it is done in the moment, and some of those moments can happen in creative coaching conversations. My main ambition in writing this chapter is to act as a *dialogue guide* and coach (Stelter, 2019), with you, dear reader, as a *dialogue partner* and client. We are about to embark on a co-creative coaching partnership. Welcome!

A note on terminology and abbreviations

I use the term client rather than coachee to refer to the person working with a coach in one-to-one, team or group contexts. Although the term coachee is used in coaching literature (e.g., Passmore & Lai, 2020), I use client because it feels less prescriptive and passive. Regarding abbreviations, professional and healthcare literature uses acronyms to abbreviate particular roles, for example, executive nurse director (END) and therapeutic radiographer (TR), and practices such as advanced practice (AP) and interprofessional collaborative practice (ICPC). Similarly, management processes such as quality improvement (QI) and total quality management (TQM), and approaches to education like interprofessional education (IPE) and health professions education (HPE) are also often abbreviated. While these might simply be an extension of the extensive use of acronyms in healthcare, I don't use them in order to avoid confusion and appeal to a wide readership. Acronyms may not be universally agreed/understood across global health systems and professions, they can alienate those 'not in the know' and writing that is overflowing with acronyms can be cumbersome to read.

Nevertheless, use of acronyms is not unusual in science disciplines and writing, including my own discipline of psychology (Hales et al., 2017). Nor are coaching and coaching psychology immune to the pervasive use of acronyms to summarise components of coaching models, leading Weinberg (2022, p. 77) to comment wryly 'the ability to develop an acronym ... seems to be an essential skill for a coach.' He suggests that coaching models that use acronyms have more in common with marketing tools than scientific models, which are better described as conceptual frameworks. Therefore, in writing this chapter, I use the term framework(s) to describe key constructs and concepts, the relationships between them and ways they can be applied in practice. I have also followed American Psychological Association (2020, p. 172) guidance that 'writing is generally easier to understand when most words are written out [in full].'

Learning outcomes

After reading and engaging with material in this chapter I hope you will be able to:

- Appreciate the value and benefits of coaching to promote advanced practice, leadership development and interprofessional collaborative practice in healthcare teams.

- Understand the psychology of leadership from the perspective of neuroscience and emotion regulation systems of threat, drive and soothing.
- Consider the relevance of systems-psychodynamic thinking and coaching to help recognise and address unconscious dynamics, processes and defences in individuals, teams and organisations.
- Critically reflect upon your own influencing skills, assumptions and ability to lead and manage with political awareness.

I suggest that you engage with these outcomes not as a tick box list, but as an *iterative, ongoing process of learning*. With some outcomes and content, you may feel confident and competent and are looking for an update and fresh insights and approaches to continuous personal and professional development. While other content in the chapter may bring new learning and challenge your assumptions and thinking about unconscious processes and defences that you may (or may not!) wish to linger over.

Activities to enhance learning

At various points, as dialogue guide and coach, I will suggest that readers take a pause for thought and reflection, to notice what is/has been going on around us. They are signposted as 'Slow down and think' and start here.

Slow down and think (1): As we begin our critically reflective coaching conversation and co-created collaborative partnership, ask yourself:

- What am I hoping to achieve and learn from engaging with the material in this chapter?

I urge you to think about how you might record your reflections and learning, for example, journalling, creative writing or taking a photo with your phone. David Pearl's (2020) book *Wanderful,* and materials on the Street Wisdom website: www.streetwisdom.org/ offer ideas for creative walking practices. For example, Figure 10.2 is a photograph taken on a Street Wisdom 'walkshop' when I was looking for creative ideas for my academic writing about compassion in higher education (Waddington, 2026, in press), where I use it to illustrate the need to 'slow down and think.'

What is coaching and coaching psychology

Passmore and Lai (2020, p. 3) define coaching as a professional helping relationship and process that emphasises reciprocal actions and social-psychological perspectives. The International Society for Coaching Psychology (2023, p. 1) define coaching psychology as 'a process for enhancing wellbeing and performance in personal and professional/work domains underpinned by models of coaching [and] psychological theories and approaches.' These are the assumptions about coaching that I bring to this chapter, underpinned by the International Coaching Federation (2025) core ethical principles of: (i) equity; (ii) collaboration; (iii) humanity; and (iv) professionalism. The chapter is also based on two further assumptions. First, some readers may coach others and/or have experienced coaching themselves and understand that professional coaching is based on shared ethical principles and values, and an evidence-based/-informed approach.

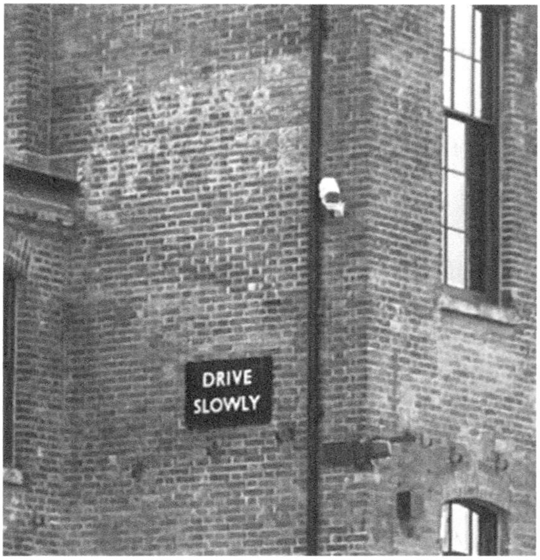

Figure 10.2 Slow down and think
Photo credit Kathryn Waddington: photograph taken at Coal Drops Yard London.

Second, some readers will be familiar with approaches such as Sir John Whitmore's GROW model – Goals, Reality, Options and Will/Way forward (Whitmore & Gaskell, 2024). This may, in some circumstances, be problematic. Susan David et al. (2013) argue that routine prescription of SMART goals – Specific, Measurable, Achievable, Relevant and Time-bound – can be difficult for neurodivergent people who may struggle with executive functioning skills. These are the cognitive skills that help us plan, organise and manage our thoughts and actions. Neurodivergent people may feel overwhelmed by having to break down goals into smaller tasks, and a more flexible approach to goal setting is needed (Doyle & McDowall, 2024).

Clutterbuck and Spence (2016) note that while goal-setting approaches (e.g., the GROW model) do have a role, they are often used in a linear, transactional manner, focusing on short-term goals. This is 'coaching by numbers,' which like 'painting by numbers' represents a pre-designed approach that is uncreative and unsuitable to the changing nature of leadership in complex healthcare systems. While a specific focus on goals and boosting a person's skills and performance is relevant in some areas (e.g., sports coaching), in professional coaching this can reflect and reinforce a deficit approach and feelings of inadequacy. Transformational coaching on the other hand goes deeper by addressing underlying beliefs, values and mindset to create meaningful long-term change (Stelter, 2019).

However, it is naïve to assume that coaching can be conducted in a completely 'goal-free' manner; clients can only live their lives in a direction that helps them move towards positive future scenarios. Drake (2015), writing from the standpoint of narrative coaching as a way of bringing new stories to life, argues it is more meaningful to work with *intentions*. Intentions involve 'setting a clear direction and the resolve to take an action or achieve an outcome [emphasis added] – without the necessity of an ultimate goal or a defined path' (p. 194). This is a better starting point for coaching; intentions are broad enough to capture the short- and long-term objectives, and clear enough to permit more specific goal-setting where/if this appears to be useful. Adopting a narrative approach is also a characteristic of Stelter's (2014; 2019) third-generation coaching, which is the core coaching framework adopted in this chapter.

Third-generation coaching

Third-generation coaching focuses on the coach and client in a narrative collaborative partnership. This differs from first-generation coaching based on a problem/goal perspective, and second-generation coaching based on a strengths-based approach. Stelter's third-generation narrative approach is framed as a developmental dialogue and, importantly, a co-creative process between coach and client. Third-generation coaching has a less goal-oriented agenda but brings a much more profound and sustainable focus on values, where coach and client create something together. They generate meaning together in dialogue, where both parties are on a journey, and where new stories gradually take shape based on:

- Appreciation and focusing on strengths and possibilities.
- Reflection on values, aspirations, wishes and dreams.
- Externalising conversations, re-authoring and telling the story in a different way.

The purpose of third-generation coaching is to offer space for reflection where coach and client find meaning together. This is less about the client finding the answer within *themselves*, but rather, within the *coaching interaction and dialogue*. This is what is meant by 'externalising conversations' where the issue is not about the client as a person but about something external to them. The client gives the issue a name (e.g., 'my frustration with ...') and then tells their story of what 'my frustration with ...' looks like from a 'bigger picture' viewpoint. This is a way of re-framing and offering new perspectives, insights and alternative ways of looking at the issue. The *values focus* of third-generation coaching is particularly pertinent to advanced practice in healthcare, acting as a guiding principle to help us organise our personal and professional lives:

> Values are somehow timeless and universal, but they have to be based on customs and events in our local communities [and areas of practice]. The ultimate goal is to facilitate and prepare leadership, communication and co-operation, not by focusing on specific goals, but by reflecting on key values as important landmarks for navigating in life.
>
> (Stelter, 2014, p. 54)

Slow down and think (2): Before we move to the next section, which explores frameworks for advanced practice:

- Take some time to reflect on your own personal and professional values.

The Values in Action Institute on Character offers a free online strengths profile to get you started: www.viacharacter.org/. It is a scientifically validated survey instrument which enables you to reflect on your 'Top 5' signature strengths. In the spirit of sharing my own assumptions and values as your dialogue guide and coach, my 'Top 5' strengths are: (i) honesty; (ii) creativity; (iii) love of learning; (iv) hope; and (v) bravery. I strongly believe in writing that exposes and explores gaps in practice and tells it as it is (Waddington, 2016a; 2024).

Frameworks for advanced practice

NHS England's (2025) multi-professional framework for advanced practice now reaches beyond previous settings and clinical focus, making a difference in areas like primary care, rehabilitation, diagnostics and justice:

> Advanced practitioners from a wide variety of professional backgrounds – nurses, midwives, allied health professionals, pharmacists, clinical scientists, optometrists, and *practitioner psychologists* [emphasis added] – are improving patient care, bridging gaps in services, and supporting sustainable, patient-focused healthcare.
> (p. 3)

Practitioner coaching psychologists are advanced practitioners in their own right and rightly belong in the above definition. We work at doctoral level (Quality Assurance Agency level 8) and are able to 'conceptualise, design and implement projects for the generation of significant new knowledge and/or understanding in coaching psychology' (British Psychological Society, 2022, p. 5). This is similar to the Royal College of Nursing's (2025) professional framework advanced level of practice and working as a consultant nurse, which also requires demonstration of doctoral-level capabilities.

Advanced practice is also about more than multi-professional frameworks. It requires true interprofessional collaboration to break down silo mentalities and tackle unequal power dynamics. The Interprofessional Education Collaborative (2023) identify core competencies for interprofessional collaborative practice:

Values and ethics: work with team members to maintain a climate of shared values, ethical conduct and mutual respect.

Role and responsibilities: use the knowledge of one's own role and team members' expertise to address individual and population health outcomes.

Communication: communicate in a responsive, responsible, respectful and compassionate manner with team members.

Teams and teamwork: apply values and principles of the science of teamwork to adapt one's own role in a variety of team settings.

I believe the field of coaching has much to offer the interprofessional practice agenda in healthcare. The British Psychological Society's Professional Standard 5 requires coaching psychologists to 'communicate effectively and bring psychological influence to bear; for example, through consultancy, training or leadership, and by working effectively with other professionals [emphasis added]' (British Psychological Society, 2022, p. 13). Leadership (and leadership coaching) is a core and unifying pillar of advanced practice and requires an understanding of the psychology of leadership.

The psychology of leadership

The current business of healthcare and public sector reform demands that leaders must relentlessly run ever-improving, reliable, high-quality services. Sustaining quality improvement initiatives is recognised as challenging; influenced by a range of contextual factors including organisational culture and leadership, individual skills and capabilities (Coles et al., 2020). Leaders are faced with the task of influencing others to do things which they may not want to do, something which requires them to change, or to behave in different ways. Leadership success is expected but elusive. Kate Pearlman-Shaw (2025) argues that today's leaders are in a double bind; a psychological concept that describes situations where we are confronted with two irreconcilable demands at the same time. Her book: *The Psychology of Effective Leadership: This Works* is an ideal companion to this chapter for readers wishing to know more about the neuroscience of leadership. It also contains tools and techniques to influence and manage through change, increasing engagement and decreasing resistance.

While leaders can be passionately committed to their profession and organisation's values and purpose, they are often overwhelmed by what they must deal with on a daily basis. For example:

> The biggest challenge for me personally is that when, as executive nurse I have to be able to present and talk and have a narrative around many issues that I don't always have the detail of. I can't always have all of the detail so that's been my biggest personal challenge.
>
> (Kelly et al., 2023, p. 3817)

Understanding the psychology of leadership from a neuroscience perspective using Paul Gilbert's (2014) drive, threat and soothing emotion regulation systems can help understand the challenges of feeling overwhelmed. All three systems have evolved for a purpose, but if the wrong system is activated at the wrong time it can derail the best-intentioned leader. Feeling overwhelmed happens when there is an imbalance between the systems, primarily associated with under-development of the soothing system.

The drive system

This system is goal-focused, its purpose is to motivate us towards resources and 'get things done' and it is associated with feelings of pursuing, progressing and achieving. It is fuelled by the release of dopamine to activate reward systems that maintain motivation. However, an over-reliance on the drive system can lead to stress, anxiety and burnout, especially if externally generated goals, in other words targets, are unrealistic. The 'drive slowly' message (Figure 10.2 above) is timely here. An obsession with targets, efficiency and prioritising short-term gains over longer-term wellbeing is risky, offering temporary 'quick wins' that mask and fail to address underlying issues/problems. This can result in professional and team cultures characterised by a 'getting high on getting by' workaholic mentality and perverse pride in the ability to cope with unrealistic demands. Attitudes towards staff who experience (and admit to) stress and burnout are often expressed in terms like 'if you can't stand the heat get out of the kitchen.' And in the 'ain't it awful' horror stories that circulate and spread as gossip, but which contain overlooked information and early warnings of systemic failures and poor practice (O'Connor et al., 2018; Waddington, 2016b).

The threat system

This emotion regulation system is fuelled by adrenalin and cortisol and tends to dominate. It evolved initially to detect and protect us from external physical threat in the environment, activating the fight, flight or freeze response. Today, this response functions to detect and protect against psychological threats in the workplace, such as perceived failure, humiliation and harms caused by destructive and abusive leadership behaviours. Webster et al. (2014) use the term toxic leadership to describe behaviours that include intimidating, bullying, manipulating (which can be mis-interpreted as influencing) and micromanaging. Their mixed-method research study with individuals who had worked with/for a toxic leader found fight, flight or freeze was a high-level coping strategy. Conversely, a leader who has a threat-driven work ethic may be constantly worried about making mistakes, which in team/organisational cultures lacking in psychological safety may lead to them working harder/longer hours, which then activates their drive system. Psychological safety is crucial here; this is the shared belief that it is safe to speak up about concerns and admit mistakes without fear of blame or reprisal (Grailey et al., 2021). Absence of psychological safety results in gossip, where concerns about patient care, poor leadership practice and systemic failures go underground and unreported (Waddington, 2012; 2021).

The soothing system

Gilbert (2014) discusses the soothing system as another configuration of emotions which is not based on the activation systems of doing and achieving (drive), nor fleeing and fighting (threat). In evolutionary terms, this is a care-giving system which operates naturally when there are no threats to defend against and no goals that must be pursued. This system taps into feel-good neurochemicals such as oxytocin, endorphins and opiates; unlike the threat and drive systems which *activate* us, the soothing system *deactivates* us. It is associated with peaceful states and feelings of being calm, content and most importantly safe. These emotional responses are linked to affiliation and collaboration; cultivating the spaces, time, team and organisation cultures where our internal affiliation systems can be activated is essential for emotional regulation. It also has a positive effect on wellbeing and the ability to be compassionate, which flows in three directions: (i) compassion towards others; (ii) compassion from others; and (iii) self-compassion (Haroun, 2021).

Slowdown and think (3): While provision of compassionate care to patients is of paramount importance in healthcare:

- How often do you offer compassion to colleagues, and how often do you receive a compassionate response/gesture from colleagues?

Lown et al. (2016) argue that provision of compassionate, collaborative care is a crucial aspect of effective interprofessional practice; yet the values and skills associated with this approach are not routinely taught, role modelled and assessed in learning and practice. Interprofessional collaborative practice and leadership can be experienced by healthcare professionals as an emotional minefield, dominated by overactive threat emotion regulation systems, particularly in the boardroom. For example, in the professional context of nursing and executive nursing leadership, Sally Bassett's (2024) doctoral research found:

> Nursing does not speak for itself, meaning that executive nurses must first establish themselves as credible to be influential within the boardroom, in contrast to medicine, which assumes a higher status ... To succeed, the executive nurse must navigate and be able to contend with the barriers, unconscious bias and prejudices associated with nursing and nurses articulated as *'nursism'* through Fricker's (2007) concept of epistemic injustice.
>
> (pp. 3–4, original emphasis)

Epistemic injustice is harm done to a person in their capacity as a knower, by undermining their capacity to engage in epistemic practices like sharing knowledge with others. It typically arises when their voice is not listened to or taken as seriously as it deserves to be taken. Unconscious bias and prejudice can be better understood and tackled by exploring the psychology of interprofessional practice (this term is used interchangeably with interprofessional collaborative practice) using insights from systems-psychodynamic thinking.

The psychology of interprofessional practice: Systems-psychodynamic thinking

Systems-psychodynamic thinking is an important field of social science, the boundaries of which are continually being refined, re-defined and researched (Sher & Lawler, 2022). It offers insights into unconscious processes and emotions experienced when working in groups and teams, which function as a protection against anxiety and threats to self-esteem. Isobel Menzies' (1960) classic paper on the structure of a hospital nursing service: 'A case-study in the functioning of social systems as a defence against anxiety' has almost iconic status in system-psychodynamic thinking and coaching (Sher & Lawler, 2022; Vesey, 2021). Anxiety in nursing work arises through contact with patients; social systems evolve as a defence in order to manage and contain this 'to-be-expected' anxiety. In Menzies' study defensive techniques included: (i) splitting up the nurse–patient relationship and ritualistic performance of tasks; (ii) depersonalisation and denial of the importance of the individual; (iii) detachment and denial of feelings; and (iv) resistance to change. While the organisation of nursing work has changed since 1960, the emotional impact of the 'to-be-expected' anxiety on nursing and allied health professions endures. This is intensified by the prevalence of dysfunctional toxic leadership and cultures in healthcare organisations and regulatory bodies.

For example, a review of cardiac surgery in England commissioned by the hospital found a persistent toxic atmosphere, dysfunctional teams, tribal-like activity and rivalry between surgeons (NHS, 2018). The Nursing and Midwifery Council (2024) commissioned an independent review into internal concerns around a toxic work environment, management practices and 'bullying, racism, incompetence and a dysfunctional workplace culture' (p. 7). The financial cost of bullying and harassment to the NHS in England (based on sickness absence costs, employee turnover, diminished productivity, compensation, litigation and industrial relations costs) was *conservatively estimated* to cost the tax payer £2,281 billion per annum (Kline & Lewis, 2018).

Unfortunately, there is overwhelming evidence of toxicity in healthcare organisations, which begins with tolerating dysfunctional behaviours, and spreads when this becomes normalised into the culture. Toxic organisations overflow with omnipotence, hubris and apathy (Hetrick, 2023), and defences and denial are alive and well in today's healthcare settings. Fortunately, systems-psychodynamic thinking shines a light on individual and collective unconscious defences (e.g., avoiding conflict, denial), and can be used in coaching to help create positive conditions that change the dynamics of a work system in a more effective and sustainable way.

Systems-psychodynamic coaching

Systems-psychodynamic coaching provides a framework for developmental and psychologically focused reflection and learning opportunities to gain insight into how 'task and organisational performance are influenced by both conscious and unconscious behaviour' (Sher & Lawler, 2022, p. 93). This type of coaching explores how the following behavioural constructs are manifest in the client's work and life:

Anxiety: is about fear of the future and can act either as a driving force or a paralysing force in professional and interprofessional relationships.
Task: is the basic constituent of work, often defined as 'primary task' which can be derailed if anxiety is not contained, resulting in anti-task behaviours to deflect free-floating anxiety.
Role: is the indicator of the boundary between professional role(s), the organisation and the external environment and stakeholders.
Authority: is the formal and official right to perform a task, authorised from above (the organisation, manager, leader), laterally (from colleagues), from below (subordinates) and from within (self-authority).
Boundaries: boundaries promote containment, provide predictability and security; task, time and territory are boundaries which need maintaining and adjusting according to changing contexts.
Identity: is about the ways clients feel and think about themselves, the way others think about them and the influence of these identities on behaviour and organisational culture.

Consider the scenario in Box 10.1, which illustrates the unconscious interplay of the above constructs and how a sub-narrative of fear and anxiety can appear in meetings.

A systems-psychodynamic coach has a number of options when working with executive teams, for example, by asking:

- Has the team defined and agreed upon its primary task?
- How does the team's ways of working contribute towards its primary task?
- How might the team engage differently with the task in hand?

Box 10.1 The unconscious at work in meetings

You are sitting in an executive meeting discussing a difficult issue that has been presented to the meeting on countless previous occasions without arriving at a resolution. Each member of the executive has a different interest in the issue, and often those interests are in competition with each other. Stalemate is reached and rather than a decision being made, the issue is postponed for discussion to a later meeting, delegated to another group or simply dropped off the agenda, leaving those involved in the preparation of the proposal feeling bruised and disempowered.

Source: Sher and Lawler (2022, pp. 99–100).

This can be followed up with one-to-one coaching focussing on the dynamics of power and control, envy, jealousy and rivalry. Individual and executive team coaching can enhance board effectiveness and improve understanding of the underlying dynamics that block decision-making.

Language and power

Language and power are really important, particularly regarding authority, role and identity. The title given to a person in a professional role gives some indication of power and authority. For example 'consultant,' 'director' and 'lead' imply a mix of authority and power; in contrast, 'coordinator' suggests that the person can only take a decision/action if everyone agrees. This can result in failures of accountability, responsibility without control and stress, as there is often little power and authority to exert influence when tasks are not achieved and targets are not met. This can trigger an ego 'threat' response, anxiety and defensive attitudes and behaviours. Ego is about a person's sense of self and includes their identity, thoughts, and feeling of self-importance and can be understood beyond the level of the individual to encompass professional and organisational egos. From an executive coaching perspective, Ratson (2024) identifies common problems associated with ego:

Overestimated ego: problems with an inflated ego leads to self-centredness, superiority, lack of compassion, arrogance, conflicts and difficult relationships.

Delicate ego: a fragile ego is easily injured and overly sensitive to criticism, judgement and failure, leading to self-doubt and insecurity.

Identity attachment: the ego forms attachments to particular identities, such as roles, positions and achievements which can be rigid and resistant to change.

Slow down and think (4): Take a moment to re-read this section on systems-psychodynamic coaching, and then focus your attention on the last section:

- I want you to think *beyond* individual egos – are any of the above ego problems manifest in your own profession, interprofessional team/s and/or organisation?

For example, Foronda et al.'s (2016) integrative review of interprofessional communication amongst healthcare professionals found that nurses in particular struggled with best practices in communication: 'due to the hierarchical structure, *egos, fear of humiliation* [emphasis added], and feeling like their opinion is not valued' (p. 39). This chimes with Sally Bassett's (2024) use of the term 'nursism' to describe negative professional stereotypes that prevent the voice of nursing being heard in the boardroom. Similarly, Kelly et al.'s (2023) research suggested that nursing 'suffered from a form of low self-esteem, even at executive level, so that nursing had also failed to be influential enough at the national platform' (p. 3818).

> Without doubt there are power rivalries and tensions. The medical director may, in fact, be the sole source of support to the executive nurse due to values alignment around altruism, serving patients and the public. The greater challenge may come from the managerial professions for example chief executives and finance directors,where there is arguably a difference in values alignment. The power of this group is greater than the power held by executive nurses, as finance dominates.
>
> (S. Bassett, personal communication, November 13, 2025)

In order for nurses and allied health professionals to get their voices heard, they need to lead, manage and influence with political awareness.

Influencing with political awareness: An interprofessional practice perspective

Hartley et al. (2013) developed a framework for political awareness based on research with managers in the UK, Australia and New Zealand, in a variety of organisations and sectors (public, voluntary and private). They used focus groups, survey and interviews to determine skills required to lead and manage with political awareness (Figure 10.3).

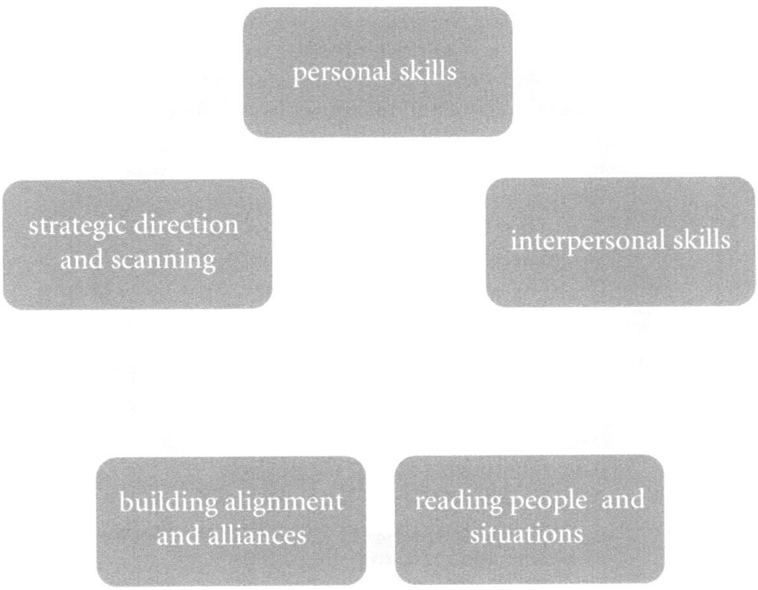

Figure 10.3 Framework for political awareness
Source: Adapted from Hartley et al. (2013, p. 18).

Personal skills of self-awareness and a proactive, rather than passive, disposition and interpersonal skills of empathy and emotional intelligence help build good working relationships at many levels. Strategically, however, reading people and situations, building alignment and alliances and strategic direction and scanning are essential influencing attributes and skills (Table 10.1).

Slow down and think (5): Looking at the dimensions of political awareness in Table 10.1 (you might want to print it, fold it up and keep it close as an aide memoir!):

- Where are your strengths, and what areas do you need to develop?
- Who are your leadership role models (these could be at work, a character in a book, a politician ....) and why did you choose them?
- What are the attributes they display and why do they reflect your views of an effective politically aware leader?

My own leadership role model is Jacinda Ardern, former New Zealand prime minister, for her humanity, compassion and, most recently, courage to step down when she knew she was experiencing burnout and had 'nothing left in the tank.' Academic analysis of her resignation speech highlights the legacy she leaves for the practice of kindness, authenticity and self-care in professional leadership (Coffe, 2023).

Table 10.1 Dimensions of Political Awareness

Reading people and situations	Recognising diversity and differences and shaping them into collaborative action Actively seeking out new alliances and partnerships rather than relying on those already in existence Ability to bring difficult issues into the open Knowing when to exclude particular interests Creating useful and realistic consensus over 'one size fits all' solutions
Building alignment and alliances	Positive leadership and management attributes Clear communication strategies and structures Active listening to identify areas of consensus Sharing resources and information Creating a supportive team climate Clarity of vision Respect and understanding of roles and responsibilities Understanding and working proactively with power dynamics
Strategic direction and scanning	Thinking long-term and having a road map of the journey Not diverted by short-term pressures Attention to what is over the horizon Analytical capacity to think through scenarios of possible futures Noticing small changes which may herald bigger shifts in practice Analysing and managing uncertainty Keeping options open rather than reaching for premature decisions

Source: Adapted from Hartley et al. (2013, p. 18).

Coaching case study

This hypothetical case study is an assimilation of material from Sher and Lawler's (2022) *An Introduction to Systems Psychodynamics: Consultancy Research and Training*. Fran (pseudonym) is a senior leader in healthcare, stepping into a highly visible and demanding role, supported by an eight-month coaching programme designed around four key areas:

(1) *Confidence in leadership voice*: overcoming self-doubt and negative professional stereotypes and stepping fully into their leadership role.
(2) *Strategic influence and interprofessional collaboration*: engaging effectively with senior leaders in other professions.
(3) *Communicating with impact*: speaking assertively and with influence in the boardroom.
(4) *Emotional regulation:* remaining calm and authoritative under pressure and role modelling compassionate leadership and self-compassion.

Coaching approach

Fran worked with their coach Harri (pseudonym) using a narrative co-creative approach underpinned by principles of systems-psychodynamics. Harri's primary task in working with Fran was to help them bring into conscious awareness things they had previously been unaware of using Socratic coaching questions (Ferris, 2024). For example:

- What assumptions are we making here?
- What are you assuming that is preventing you from stepping forward?
- Where is the evidence to support your assumptions?
- What are the implications and consequences of these assumptions?
- What power dynamics are going on that you are getting caught up in?
- What would be the most 'un-Fran like' thing you could do in that situation?

Themes and insights

Coaching helped Fran recognise they had earned their place in the boardroom and could contribute meaningfully without needing to dominate or becoming defensive or passive-aggressive in their behaviour. They appreciated the value of the role of coaching in promoting wellbeing and the importance of self-compassion and being kind to yourself as a way of 'switching on' their soothing emotion regulation system. Fran began to approach high-stakes meetings with calmness, increasingly drawing on interprofessional collaboration and external expertise to broaden their influence. Fran reported that coaching provided a psychologically safe space to voice concerns, build confidence and demonstrate impact and influence in a highly visible senior leadership role.

Concluding with self-compassion

We are coming to the end of our coaching journey in this chapter, and I would like to thank you for making it this far with me in my attempt to write differently. I would also like to leave you with the gift of self-compassion as a coaching tool to help you become a more effective leader and role model for the people you lead and influence. Self-compassion is about being supportive towards yourself when experiencing suffering or stress, whether caused by personal mistakes and inadequacies or external life challenges. Kristin Neff's (2023) theoretical model of self-compassion comprises: (i) increased self-kindness; (ii) common humanity; (iii) mindfulness; and (iv) reduced self-judgement, isolation and overidentification. Useful resources, practices and self-compassion exercises, such as changing your critical self-talk, can be found on her website (Neff, 2025). I also hope you are able to use some of the theoretical aspects of the psychology of leadership and application of systems-psychodynamic thinking to help you navigate your advanced practice journey and influence positive change. Finally, I am curious as to where your engagement with the material in the chapter might take you next?

Slow down and think (6): As we end our critically reflective coaching conversation, ask yourself:

- If we were able to speak to each other three years from now, what would you tell me about how your professional life has evolved, and how you used your learning from this chapter to influence others?

My answer to you, in this hypothetical future conversation, would be that I have been able to influence interprofessional practice in healthcare in a small way through ripple effects from this chapter, and have strengthened my identity as a creative writer and coach.

Acknowledgements

I would like to thank Dr Sally Bassett and Professor Annie Topping for their helpful thoughts and comments on an earlier version of this chapter.

References

Adsit, J. (2025). *Writing and health care: Creative and critical approaches*. Bloomsbury Academic.

American Psychological Association. (2020). *Publication manual of the American Psychological Association* (7th ed.). American Psychological Association.

Bassett, S. (2024). *Perspectives and explanations of successful executive nurse leadership in English NHS Trust Boards*. Oxford Brookes University. https://radar.brookes.ac.uk/radar/items/07ab31a6-c242-444e-a5ae-ea02765e4fc7/1

Boncori, I. (2022). Writing the personal. In M. Kostera (Ed.), *How to write differently: A quest for meaningful academic writing*. Edward Elgar Publishing.

British Psychological Society. (2022). *Level 8 standards for coaching psychology*. www.bps.org.uk/member-networks/division-coaching-psychology

Clutterbuck, D., & Spence, G. B. (2016). Working with goals in coaching. In T. Bachkirova, G. Spence & D. Drake (Eds.), *The SAGE handbook of coaching* (pp. 221–239). Sage.

Coffe, H. (2023, January 20). Jacinda Ardern: The 'politics of kindness' is a lasting legacy. *The Conversation*. https://theconversation.com/jacinda-ardern-the-politics-of-kindness-is-a-lasting-legacy-198186

Coles, E., Anderson, J., Maxwell, M., Harris, F. M., Gray, N. M., Milner, G. M., & MacGillivray, S. (2020). The influence of contextual factors on healthcare quality improvement initiatives: A realist review. *Systematic Reviews, 9*(94), 1–22. https://doi.org/10.1186/s13643-020-01344-3

David, S., Clutterbuck, D., & Megginson, D. (Eds.). (2013). *Beyond goals: Effective strategies for coaching and mentoring*. Routledge.

Doyle, N., & McDowall, A. (2024). *Neurodiversity coaching: A psychological approach to supporting neurodivergent talent and career potential.* Routledge.

Drake, D. B. (2015). *Narrative coaching: Bringing our new stories to life.* CNC Press.

Edelist, T., Friesen, F., Ng, S., Fernandez, N., Bélisle, M., Lechasseur, K., Rochette, A., Vachon, B., & Caty, M-E. (2024). Critical reflection in team-based practice: A narrative review. *Medical Education in Review, 58,* 1166–1177. https://doi.org/10.1111/medu.15462

Ferris, S. P. (2024, November 19). Ancient answers: Socratic dialogue's role in executive coaching. *International Coaching Federation.* https://coachingfederation.org/blog/ancient-answers-socratic-dialogues-role-in-executive-coaching/

Foronda, C., MacWilliams, B., & McArthur, E. (2016). Interprofessional communication in healthcare: An integrative review. *Nurse Education in Practice, 19,* 36–40. https://dx.doi.org/10.1016/j.nepr.2016.04.005

Fricker, M. (2007). *Epistemic injustice: Power and the ethics of knowing.* Oxford University Press.

Gilbert, P. (2014). The origins and nature of compassion focused therapy. *British Journal of Clinical Psychology, 53,* 6–41. https://doi.org/10.1111/bjc.12043

Grailey, K. E., Murray, E., Reader, T., & Brett, S. J. (2021). The presence and potential impact of psychological safety in the healthcare setting: An evidence synthesis. *BMC Health Services Research, 21*(773), 1–15. https://doi.org/10.1186/s12913-021-06740-6

Hales, A. H., Williams, K. D., & Rector, J. (2017, January 31). Alienating the audience: How abbreviations hamper scientific communication. *Association for Psychological Science.* www.psychologicalscience.org/observer/alienating-the-audience-how-abbreviations-hamper-scientific-communication

Haroun, J. (2021). Flourishing in the university: Could compassion help? In K. Waddington (Ed.), *Towards the compassionate university, From golden thread to global impact.* Taylor & Francis (pp. 102–118).

Hartley, J., Alford, J., Hughes, O., & Yates, S. (2013). *Leading with political astuteness: A white paper.* Chartered Management Institute.

Hetrick, S. (2023). *Toxic organizational cultures and leadership: How to build and sustain a healthy workplace.* Routledge.

Hunaiti, Z. (2024). Empowering healthcare headers: Coaching for leadership development. *Encyclopedia, 4,* 1752–1759. www.mdpi.com/2673-8392/4/4/115

International Coaching Federation. (2025). *ICF code of ethics.* https://coachingfederation.org/credentialing/coaching-ethics/icf-code-of-ethics/

International Society for Coaching Psychology. (2023). *What is coaching psychology?* www.isfcp.info/what-is-coaching-psychology/

Interprofessional Education Collaborative. (2023). *IPEC core competencies.* www.ipecollaborative.org/ipec-core-competencies

Kelly, D., Horseman, Z., Strachan, F. E., Hamilton, S., Jones, A., Holloway, A., Rafferty, A. M., Noble, H., Reid, J., Harris, R., & Smith, P. (2023). Strengthening the role of the executive nurse director: A qualitative interview study. *Journal of Advanced Nursing, 79*(10), 3809–3823. https://doi.org/10.1111/jan.15699

Kline, R., & Lewis, D. (2018) The price of fear: Estimating the financial cost of bullying and harassment to the NHS in England. *Public Money & Management, 39*(3), 166–174. https://doi.org/10.1080/09540962.2018.1535044

Lown, B. A., McIntosh, S., Gaines, M. E., McGuinn, K., & Hatem, D. S. (2016). Integrating compassionate, collaborative care (the "triple C") into health professional education to advance the triple aim of health care. *Academic Medicine, 91*(3), 310–316. https://doi.org/10.1097/ACM.0000000000001077

Menzies, I. E. P. (1960). A case-study in the functioning of social systems as a defence against anxiety. A report on a study of the nursing service of a general hospital. *Human Relations, 13*(2), 95–121.

Neff, K. (2023). Self-compassion: Theory, method, research and intervention. *Annual Review of Psychology, 74,* 193–218. https://doi.org/10.1146/annurev-psych-032420-031047

Neff, K. (2025). *Self-compassion practices*. https://self-compassion.org/self-compassion-practices/
NHS. (2018, August 9). Cardiac surgery at St Georges – updated statement. www.stgeorges.nhs.uk/newsitem/cardiac-surgery-at-st-georges-updated-statement-thursday-9-august-2018/
NHS England. (2025). *Multi-professional framework for advanced practice 2025*. https://advanced-practice.hee.nhs.uk/multi-professional-framework-for-advanced-practice/
Nursing and Midwifery Council/Rise Associates. (2024). *The Nursing and Midwifery Council independent culture review*. https://riseassociates.co.uk/news/nazir-afzal-and-rise-associates-launch-nmc-independent-culture-review/
O'Connor, N., Kotze, B., & Storm, V. (2018). What's to be done when 'foul whisperings are abroad'? Gossip and rumour in health organisations. *Australasian Psychiatry, 26*(1), 30–33. https://doi.org/10.1177/1039856217716292
Passmore, J., & Lai, Y-L. (2020). Coaching psychology: Exploring definitions and research contribution to practice. In J. Passmore & D. Tee (Eds.), *Coaching researched: A coaching psychology reader* (pp. 3–22). Wiley.
Pearl, D. (2020). *Wanderful: Find wonder in the everyday every day*. Unbound.
Pearlman-Shaw, K. (2025). *The psychology of effective leadership: This works*. Routledge.
Ratson, M. (2024, March 21). The challenge of the ego and taking things personally. *Psychology Today*. www.psychologytoday.com/gb/blog/the-wisdom-of-anger/202403/the-challenge-of-the-ego-and-taking-things-personally
Robson, I. (2022). *The reflective leader: Reflexivity in practice*. Emerald Publishing Limited.
Royal College of Nursing. (2025). Levels for the registered nurse. www.rcn.org.uk/Professional-Development/Levels-of-nursing
Sher, M., & Lawler, D. (2022). *An introduction to systems psychodynamics: Consultancy research and training*. Routledge.
Stelter, R. (2014). Third generation coaching: Reconstructing dialogues through collaborative practice and a focus on values. *International Coaching Psychology Review, 9*(1), 51–66. https://doi.org/10.53841/bpsicpr.2014.9.1.51
Stelter, R. (2019). *The art of dialogue in coaching: Towards transformative change*. Routledge.
Vesey, R. (2021, January 20). The depth and breadth of the matter: Five tips for systems-psychodynamic executive coaching. Tavistock Consulting. https://tavistockconsulting.co.uk/insight/the-depth-and-breadth-of-the-matter-five-tips-for-systems-psychodynamic-coaching/
Waddington, K. (2012). *Gossip and organizations*. Routledge.
Waddington, K. (2016a). The compassion gap in UK universities. *International Practice Development Journal, 6*(1), Article 10. https://doi.org/10.19043/ipdj.61.010
Waddington, K. (2016b). Rethinking gossip and scandal in healthcare organizations. *Journal of Health Organization and Management, 30*(6), 810–817. https://doi.org/10.1108/JHOM-03-2016-0053
Waddington, K. (2021). *Gossip, organization and work: A research overview*. Routledge.
Waddington, K. (2024). Beyond bullshit: Writing with compassion, clarity and creativity. *The Psychologist*, August/September. www.bps.org.uk/psychologist/beyond-bullshit-writing-compassion-clarity-and-creativity
Waddington, K. (2026, in press). *How to be a compassionate academic: Scholarship and sustainable development*. Edward Elgar Publishing.
Waddington, K., & Jones, S. (2023). Action learning and coaching as an integrated approach for supporting women's career development. *Journal of Perspectives in Applied Academic Practice, 11*(2), 90–108. https://doi.org/10.56433/jpaap.v11i2.548
Webster, V., Brough, P., & Daly, K. (2014). Fight, flight or freeze: Common responses for follower coping with toxic leadership. *Stress and Health, 32*(4), 346–354. https://doi.org/10.1002/smi.2626
Weinberg, J. (2022). Does coaching psychology have status anxiety? *The Coaching Psychologist, 18*(2), 73–79. https://doi.org/10.53841/bpstcp.2022.18.2.73
Whitmore, J., & Gaskell, T. (2024). *Coaching for performance: The principles and practice of coaching and leadership* (6th ed.). John Murray Business.

Index

Note: Page numbers in *italics* refer to figures and **bold** refer to tables.

For Product Safety Concerns and Information please contact our EU representative GPSR@taylorandfrancis.com Taylor & Francis Verlag GmbH, Kaufingerstraße 24, 80331 München, Germany